The Definit[...] Diet for Weight Loss Surgery for Health & Healing

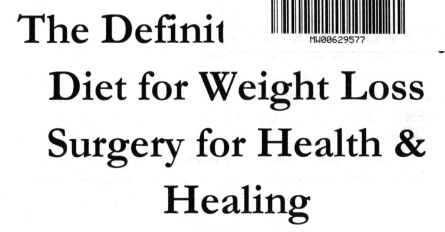

The Proven Benefits from the Alkaline Diet and Acid Reflux Diet For Gastric Sleeve Surgery & Bariatric Surgery

Dr. Jonathan Brown

Dr Patt Wright

Sarah Levine M.D.

Patt Vince Harrison

Redford E. Gordon

Table of Contents

PART 1

Introduction

The following chapters will discuss all of the many health benefits to maintaining an alkaline diet as well as the keys to unlocking all of your health potentials. We will look at the chemistry behind the pH scale and how it works and behave within our bodies. We will learn all about why an alkaline balanced diet is the best way to keep your body as healthy as possible.

Maintaining a happy and healthy body can be a real challenge, but within the pages of this book, you will find all of the secrets and tips for making an alkaline-based pH balanced diet a major part of your life with high-impact solutions and surefire methods for creating a healthy pH balance in your own body chemistry.

We will also look at some amazing meal ideas to keep you going strong on the alkaline diet all day every day. Don't miss a single meal with these new and exciting meal ideas. Never be in the dark again! After reading this book, you will know everything you need in order to create and maintain a healthy and satisfying alkaline diet.

There are plenty of books on this subject on the market, so thanks again for choosing this one! Every effort was made to ensure it is full of as much useful information as possible. Please enjoy!

Chapter 1: What is the Alkaline Diet?

We eat the foods that we eat for all kinds of different reasons. Sure, from an evolutionary standpoint, we eat food so that we can take in calories and convert them into energy in order to fuel our bodies and keep us going throughout the entire day. The food we eat also provides us with the essential nutrients that our bodies need in order to keep them running in an optimal manner.

But we also eat food for pleasure, the sheer joy of tasting something amazing that we truly love. We eat socially. Food has been a way of bringing people together since the very dawn of civilization. Sometimes we use food for comfort and sometimes we use it to mark formal and important occasions. We use food as a proving ground over which to test out new prospective romantic partners.

And yet, for all that food can do for us, so many of us take it for granted and don't seek out ways to make our food work for us. Used correctly, food and nutrition are tools that can turn our bodies into the healthiest and efficient powerhouse that nature intended them to be.

With so many different diets and nutrition plans out there, it can be hard to know which one is right for you. Well, you're reading this book so you already know that you're on the right track!

Indeed, the alkaline diet is a tried and tested way to get the most out of your body. But how does it work? Why does it work? How can eating an alkaline diet optimize your body and health?

The key to understanding the science and chemistry behind how the foods we eat affect us is to understand that just like the fundamental laws of physics, every action has an equal and opposite reaction. Or in other words, everything that we put into our bodies will affect us based on the characteristics of that particular food item. So if we eat a lot of things that cause the same or similar effects on our bodies, we can influence and even control the effects and changes that our body takes by carefully selecting the foods that we eat and what effect they have on our bodies. As the popular saying goes — you are what you eat.

To illustrate, imagine you are walking through the woods and you accidentally brush up against a poison ivy leaf. Well, sorry to say it, but there is a very good chance that you are going to develop an itchy poison ivy rash. If however, you get completely naked and roll around in an entire patch of poison ivy, you are pretty much guaranteed to get poison ivy and a whole lot of it!

Humorous examples aside, it stands to reason that if we know that a particular food or food group has a particular effect on our body, we can effectively control any number of internal body systems by carefully planning and selecting the foods we eat.

So how does the alkaline diet promote health? Well, the alkaline diet is all about balance. So many of the negative health issues in our lives are the result of an imbalance in our bodies. So much of the history of medicine revolves around finding the ideal balances for the human body.

For many, many years, doctors around the world attributed all of our health conditions, whether good or ill, to a balance or imbalance in what they referred to as the "humors". As far back as Ancient Greece and Ancient Rome, there was a near-universal belief that four humors or bodily fluids influenced every aspect of health and temperament, and ill health or ill temperament was the result of deficiencies or excesses on one or more of these four humors. These four humors were black bile, yellow bile, phlegm, and blood. Each of these four humors was associated with a particular personality type and other such characteristics.

When a person came to an ancient doctor with an ailment, the ancient doctor would examine their patient to determine their temperament and along with other factors would determine where their imbalance in humors was, and then they would come up with a treatment plan with the intention of balancing the patient's humors. So in other words, for millennia, the goal of medicine has been to achieve balance in the human body.

And while many of the theories and practices of ancient physicians have long ago fallen out of use in favor of new techniques and schools of thought, modern science has nevertheless confirmed at least some aspects of ancient medicine, namely, the concept of balance itself.

While we don't hear much about black bile, yellow bile, or phlegm anymore in modern medicine, the fourth humor that ancient doctors treated is certainly still extremely prominent in modern medicine — blood.

Blood is still very much our life force just as it was believed by ancient doctors. Blood is the fluid that keeps us living and breathing and a proper medical understanding is absolutely integral to maintain overall good health.

So how can we maintain a good balance in our blood? What aspect of our blood do we even need to balance? What negative effects can we avoid by maintaining balanced blood and what positive ones can we promote?

While those ancient doctors were certainly on the right track, they had a few key factors wrong so, in order to move forward, we are going to need a firmer and more modern grasp of the science behind our health and nutrition.

To understand this concept a little bit better, we need to understand one of the most fundamental aspects of chemistry. This integral part of chemistry and science as a whole is known as the pH balance or the pH scale. We are going to learn all about the pH balance or the pH scale and how it can affect our bodies in a positive way in the following chapters. First, we will learn what a pH balance is.

Chapter 2: What is a pH Balance?

The first thing we need to understand on our journey to the perfect internal balance via the alkaline diet is exactly just what the pH balance is. Furthermore, we need to understand how the chemical characteristics of a substance or fluid play a role in determining where it falls on the pH scale.

What exactly does the pH scale measure? In short, the pH scale is a measure of the acidity or basicity of solution in which the solvent is water. Such a solution is known as an aqueous solution. In other words, when a substance is dissolved in or is otherwise mixed with water, it can then be tested and measured on the pH scale.

An aqueous solution can be defined as either an acid or a base, as this is precisely what the pH scale is meant to determine. An aqueous solution that is basic is referred to as being alkaline. This gives us a pretty good indication of what the alkaline diet is all about. The pH scale itself is a type of scale known as a logarithmic scale. This means that each equidistant quantified measure is an order of magnitude greater than the previous measurement on the scale. The scale ranges from zero to fourteen, with a neutral pH value being in the middle at seven.

Solutions that have a pH value of less the median value of seven are defined as being acidic, while the opposite scenario, in which a solution is measured to have a pH value of higher than seven — that solution is called basic. Water that is pure and unadulterated is pH neutral which is to say that it should prove to have a pH value of seven when tested, as natural dihydrogen oxide, the chemical name for water is neither a base nor an acid. If that is not the case, then the water should be tested for impurities.

While it is possible for an aqueous solution to have a pH value greater than fourteen or less than zero, these would have to be extremely acidic or extremely basic solutions and would not only be decisively deadly to ingest and even extremely dangerous just to touch. Therefore, for practical purposes, official pH values are nearly always represented on a scale between zero and fourteen.

The pH scale is defined by a set of international standards that are determined and agreed upon by an international scientific body. There are several ways to test the pH level of an aqueous solution, with one of the most notable ones being the use of a glass electrode combined with a pH meter. This scientific instrument determines the difference between a pH electrode and a control electrode in terms of their respective electrical potential. This difference in the electrical potential of a solution relates directly to the acidity of the solution and can therefore be used to give it a standard value.

Another very popular and frequently used means by which to test the pH value of an aqueous solution is by using one of the various compounds known as pH indicators.

A pH indicator is generally some kind of substance that when mixed with an aqueous solution results in a chemical reaction that will literally change the color of the solution, and by examining and comparing the color of the resulting solution, the pH value of the solution can be determined. There are other pH indicators that indicate the pH level of a solution by chemical reactions that result in other physical indicators such as odor for example. However, by far the most common variety of pH indicators are visual in nature, generally based around color.

One of the most common types of pH indicators is the naturally occurring family of chemical compounds called anthocyanin. These compounds naturally change color reflects the pH balance of whatever item the compound is found within. Generally, these compounds are found in colored plant leaves or other plant parts. One of the most common sources of these pH indicating compounds is from the leaves of a red cabbage. The reason for this is because it is quite easy to extract anthocyanin from a red cabbage making it the perfect resource for a homemade pH indicator test for either health or educational purposes.

Anthocyanin can be found in many different plants though, such as the leaves of the aforementioned red cabbage, but also in certain flowers such as the geranium, the poppy, and also rose petals. Berries and stems can also house anthocyanin compounds such as blueberries and blackcurrants as well as rhubarb. In short, most plants or vegetables that have reddish, purplish, or bluish color in all likelihood contain at least a small amount of anthocyanin compound. When used as a pH indicator by mixing it with an aqueous solution, an anthocyanin compound will become redder the more acidic the solution is and will turn from red to purple to blue the more alkaline the solution is.

Another very commonly used pH indicator since medieval times is the substance called litmus which is derived from various species of lichen. In fact, the word litmus itself means colored moss in its original language, Old

Norse. Just like anthocyanin compounds, litmus will turn red when exposed to acidic solutions and blue when exposed to basic solutions. You may even be familiar with the term 'litmus test'. It has come to be used very commonly and very broadly as a metaphor for anything that could be used to soundly distinguish between multiple options.

So with pH balance being fundamental to the chemical nature of all kinds of biological material including the foods we eat, how do we know if and how such foods are affecting our health? We will continue learning about pH imbalance in our bodies to find out. The next chapter will go into the science of how pH balance or more specifically imbalance can affect our bodies and our health.

Chapter 3: The Science Behind pH Imbalance

Every single substance in the world has a pH balance and that includes all of us. Sure, we don't make cabbages change color when we pick them up, but our bodies must maintain a certain pH level in order to live and function properly. This pH balance that is naturally maintained in our bodies is called the acid-based balance and it is quite literally exactly what it sounds like — the balance of acidic and basic substances in your body. More specifically though, when we are referring to the acid-base balance of our bodies, we are most often referring to the pH balance of our blood.

The human body is designed with a few systems in place intended to keep the natural pH levels regulated at an appropriate balance between acidity and alkalinity. Both the kidneys as well as the lungs have a very important role to play in this process. As we previously laid out, the pH balance is generally expressed as a value between zero and fourteen, with seven being the neutral value. And remember that pure and unadulterated water should have a pH value of exactly seven. Knowing then that water is neutral seven on the pH scale, and knowing also that our bodies are designed to maintain an even pH balance, it would stand to reason that our blood should have a neutral pH value of seven as well, right?

Well, not quite. And this is a major key to understand the alkaline diet. The ideal blood pH level is not actually a neutral seven but instead generally should be about a 7.40 on the pH scale. This value can vary slightly from person to person, but that is the standard average. And yes, that's right— the human body should have a blood pH level that is a little bit on the alkaline side.

Generally speaking, it is the kidneys and lungs that regulate this pH level, so if they are not functioning normally, the blood pH level can become imbalanced. This kind of pH imbalance can lead to serious medical conditions which are called acidosis or alkalosis depending on which direction the imbalance goes in. It is important to note that these serious medical conditions must be treated by a medical professional and diet alone cannot entirely reverse these conditions.

Now, what we're talking about in this book is the small, minor imbalances that a general practitioner wouldn't be concerned about because they aren't severe enough to have a serious debilitating effect, but that certainly do have your body operating in sub-optimal conditions, and more importantly, the alkaline diet that can have it function far better than you ever imagined possible.

So in order to better understand how the alkaline diet will allow us to correct these small but important pH imbalances, we'll need to have a complete understanding of what could throw our pH out of balance and why it might happen.

As we have established a moment ago, the primary regulators of the body's pH level are the kidneys and the lungs. There are a large number of small systems in our bodies that have their own pH level and regulate them in their own ways, but the two main, body-wide regulators are the lungs and kidneys.

As you are likely already aware, we take in oxygen with our lungs when we inhale and expel carbon dioxide when we exhale. The oxygen that we take in is absorbed inside our lungs and used as fuel by our cells. The waste product that our cells produce by using the oxygen is carbon dioxide. Which is all very simple and pretty straightforward and familiar to all of us but here's the important part — carbon dioxide is slightly acidic. So by making slight adjustments to how much carbon dioxide is released or retained, our lungs are able to make adjustments to the overall acid-base level of our blood.

Similarly, the kidneys being the filtration system for the vascular system have the ability to excrete small amounts of acidic or basic compounds into the blood in order to make slight alterations to our blood chemistry. This is a slow process as compared to the more immediate effect of the lungs' pH regulatory system. So the lungs and the kidneys could be thought of as the short-term and long-term blood pH level regulators of our body.

If the blood pH level is out of balance, then it can lead to one of these two conditions — alkalosis and acidosis. With the standard balanced blood pH level being 7.40, anything below 7.35 is considered acidosis and anything above 7.45 is called alkalosis. Again, it is important to note that these are serious medical conditions and must be treated by a medical professional. It is always best to consult your doctor if you are suffering from these conditions. What we can do, however, is assist our body's natural pH regulation system by maintaining a blood pH level that is within the tolerable limits.

A low blood pH level or in other words, slightly acidic blood is far more common than the inverse and so that it is what we are primarily focusing on — an alkaline diet that will help us maintain a healthy blood pH level.

While any level measured at 7.35 and under is acidosis and needs professional medical treatment, it is far too common for our blood pH level to fall into that 'safe' range of 7.36-7.39 without being at that ideal sweet spot of 7.40. If you want to get the most out of your body, if you want your body to be operating at peak performance, and if you want to live your absolute healthiest life, then the 'safe' level of 7.36 is not tolerable for your body.

If you are truly serious about your health and your wellbeing, then the 'safe' blood pH level of 7.39 isn't even good enough for you. You need to have the absolute optimal blood pH level and you will settle for nothing but a perfect 7.40. Continue on reading in the next chapters and we are going to show you how.

Chapter 4: Why Alkaline is Best

If our body's pH level is all about balance, then why would maintaining an alkaline diet be superior to an acidic one? Shouldn't we be consuming a perfect balance of alkaline and acidic foods and nutrition? If those are among the questions you are now asking yourself, then you are on the right track. Those are great questions to ask.

There are several reasons why an alkaline diet is a crucial component in maintaining a healthy body and blood pH level. Remember that magic number? The ideal pH level for our blood that will allow our body to operate optimally? That is right — it was 7.40. And do you remember what the pH value for perfectly pure, unadulterated water is? That is right — it was a perfect seven. So what that means, of course, is that the ideal blood pH balance is in fact slightly alkaline at 0.4 units more basic than water.

So we can see already that in order to maintain our ideal pH balance, we will need to intake more alkaline foods than acidic foods. Of course, that is not to say that you can never consume anything acidic. In fact, it is important to have acids as well in order to maintain balance. We just need to be perfectly aware that our body does in fact require a slight alkaline balance and so we should be mindful of this when we plan our meals and overall diets.

This balance may also be reflected in the foods we choose to eat. They don't necessarily need to be extremely alkaline in order to transfer to us the health benefits we are looking for. They may only need to have a slight pull on the alkaline side of the scale. It all depends on our individual bodies and what they are in need of. And of course, everything scales. So a lot of a slightly alkaline substance may have the same value as a little of something with a higher alkaline value. Remember as well that the pH scale is logarithmic which is to say that each unit is exponential to the value of the previous unit. That means that consuming something with an alkaline value of nine would be ten times more alkaline than something with the alkaline value of eight. This is why we need to be careful when consuming anything that is alkaline or acidic. Things can become unhealthy or even dangerous in a real hurry. So, remember to plan ahead and do everything in moderation.

Another equally surface-level reason why it is important to consume a healthy amount of alkaline rich foods is because whether we are aware of it or not, many if not most of the foods we eat on a regular basis are either slightly or moderately acidic. Some very common foods and beverages even go as far as being highly acidic.

Now, again, it bears repeating that this does not mean that you cannot or should not consume these types of acidic foods and beverages at all. In fact, some of these acidic foods and beverages are very healthy and high in essential nutrients. The important thing, however, is to be aware of how much acidic substances we are consuming and how acidic those substances are.

Do you like fruit juices? How about coffee? Those are two great examples of highly acidic beverages that many of us consume on a regular basis. That is not necessarily a bad thing but just think about this — are you taking in the necessary amount of alkaline foods or liquids in order to maintain a healthy and optimal balance?

And what's more, it can often be a good deal more complicated than whether the particular food item that we are consuming is acidic or alkaline on a surface level. What makes the important difference is how the item we consume affects our blood pH level after it has been metabolized. And that could, in fact, be a good deal different than what it might seem to be based on the original acidity or alkalinity of the food item in question.

Another very important reason to remember to include alkaline foods in our diet in order to maintain a good acid-base blood balance is that an acid rich environment is considered by medical professionals to be a hotbed of disease and illness. And remember, it doesn't take much to become imbalanced in one's blood levels, so even a minor imbalance could quickly become a breeding ground for all manner of illness and health problems that you will absolutely want to avoid.

Just by remembering to consume a healthy and appropriate amount of alkaline foods and drinks, we can be safeguarding ourselves from any number of serious health concerns that could be lurking in our very blood. If you want to kill all of those potential illnesses dead before they become a real concern, you will need to act now and ensure that you are consuming an appropriate amount of alkaline foods.

This is the very topic that we will be going into next. We now know how important it is to maintain a good acid-base blood balance. We now know what that optimal blood pH balance is. And most importantly, we now know the dangers associated with having blood that is too acidic, and why it is so common for us to have a blood pH level that skews a little bit too acidic but not enough to go into full acidosis.

Equipped with this crucial information, we can now move on to learning about how to apply these factors to our everyday lives. Now, we are going to learn everything we need to know about how to create and maintain a balanced blood pH level, and all the tips and tricks to make it easy and straightforward.

Are you ready to have a body operating at optimal health? Are you ready to get the most out of your diet? Are you ready to prevent disease and illness that you didn't even know you were susceptible to?

Then continue on reading on, because all of your questions are about to be answered.

Chapter 5: Creating an Acid-Alkaline Balance

In this chapter, we are going to take a look at some of the biggest and best ways to gain control of your acid-alkaline blood levels and ensure that you can maintain them at an optimal level. Many of the things that we are going to talk about here are not just about diet. In fact, even the alkaline diet is not just about diet — it is about habits. It is about keeping good habits, maintaining regular health goals, and being in tune with your own body.

There are plenty of signs and symptoms that you may notice in the event that your body is too acidic. It is very likely that you will be experiencing chronic fatigue if your body is too acidic. Even if it seems that though you have been sleeping enough, you may still feel this way. Other symptoms of overly acidic blood are pain, headaches, joint pain, and stiffness.

Generally, people with acidic blood express an overall feeling of sluggishness and lethargy — sometimes even depression. It is also associated with a sense of irritability and a dulling of the mental faculties.

Obviously, if you are experiencing any of these symptoms, it will be in your best interest to correct them to the best of your ability. There are lots of ways to make your blood more alkaline and we will look at a few here.

First of all, you will want to make sure that your symptoms or feelings are in fact coming from a pH imbalance. In order to do that, you will need to check your blood pH levels regularly in order to maintain an up-to-date record of your pH levels. You can do this very easily with simple, inexpensive home testing kits available online and at many drug stores. You can get an instant and highly accurate reading and find out exactly where your body's pH balance is sitting. These simple test kits can help you make healthy and informed decisions about your personal health based on accurate and current information. This is a great, convenient, and inexpensive way to always be on top of your health.

Now, before we get into specific diet plans, let us talk about some changes that we can make to our diet in a general sense that will help improve our blood pH levels. One such thing that we can do to ensure that we are maintaining appropriate levels of acidity in our blood is by making sure that we eat more greens and dark-colored vegetables in general. Greens are not always the most popular foods to eat despite their great reputation and association with good health. But there are ways to make greens and other veggies fun and exciting and taste great.

You could try new recipes and try new types of veggies that you have never tried before. If you already love veggies, try to make sure that you get a good amount on a regular basis, if not every day. Even if you have a particular proclivity for veggies, it's easy to leave them out on occasion. Try to avoid that tendency.

And if you don't like veggies, maybe it has something to do with a reduction in their appeal on account of processed foods and excessive artificial sugars. Simply by cutting these things out of our diets as much as possible can dramatically reduce cravings for said items and make good, nutrient-rich foods like dark, green veggies far more appealing.

Either way, try to experiment with new ways of getting your veggies and making them fun and enjoyable. Try keeping some prepared in advance so that you always have a quick and healthy snack.

Here is another quick tip for general health and well-being. Every morning, the first thing you do when you wake up should be to drink a great big glass of ice-cold water as fast as you can. Why? Well, it's quick and it's easy, it costs nothing, and it has all kinds of great health and wellness benefits both short-term and long-term. First of all, the most immediate benefit is that ice-cold blast of invigorating water will snap you wide awake quicker and more effectively than any caffeinated beverage.

What's more, there's nothing better than an icy surprise to jump-start your body and kick your metabolism into a high-gear first thing in the morning. And because our friend water is completely calorie-free, that basically amounts to an energy boost and metabolism enhancer for free, metabolically speaking.

And do you want to take this brilliant life hack one step further and bring it into our alkaline friendly lifestyle? Add just a touch of lemon to that morning burst of water, or better yet, all the water you drink and you will get all the previous benefits plus that boost to your body's alkalinity that you need to function at peak efficiency. This may seem counter-intuitive given that lemon is acidic, but remember, it is not always about the acid-alkaline balance of the compound itself. It is how our bodies metabolize that compound. And lemon, being a well-known metabolism booster, will give you that alkaline push you need.

Of course, sometimes it is about the actual acidity of the food we are eating. Specifically, it is about the amount of acidic foods we are eating. If you find that you are suffering from symptoms of acid reflux, kidney stones, low bone density, or anything else associated with high body acidity levels — that is almost certainly a strong indication that you should be strictly limiting your intake of acidic foods.

This goes of course for any of the obvious culprits like tomato sauce or spicy foods, but there are some less obvious foods that metabolize into an acidic by-product in our bodies that we should be cautious of as well. This includes many processed cakes and cereals, often grain such as rice, oats or pasta, and even certain nuts like peanuts or walnuts. The key here is to just always be aware of what we are consuming and keep everything in moderation.

Beverages as well should be kept in moderation especially coffee and alcohol since both of which are associated with many negative health effects when consumed in excess, far beyond body acid-alkaline balance.

Chapter 6: Alkaline Diet for Vegetarians

Don't let the title fool you, this isn't just for vegetarians. The alkaline diet is great for anyone and everyone. If you are already a vegetarian — great, you are already in a great spot to maintain an amazing alkaline diet. If you're not a vegetarian, that's okay too. Remember in the previous chapter when we said that it is not necessarily about how acidic the foods we eat are but the quantities? Well, that goes for meat. Most meats are extremely acid forming in our bodies.

That means that while they may not be acidic to the taste or even particularly acidic on a pH test, they metabolize in our bodies into an acidic by-product. So naturally, most alkaline diet meal plans are going to be either vegan or vegetarian, or just very light on the meat and dairy. That doesn't mean, of course, that you need to completely remove meat from your diet, but if you choose to continue eating meat, you will need to be highly aware of the quality and quantity of the meat you consume. Keep it moderate and make sure to maintain good health otherwise and you should be okay.

But speaking of acid-forming diets, what so bad about them? We have seen some of the symptoms of having a seriously acidic blood pH level, but what if we're just prone to eating a little bit on the acid-forming side? Well, simply by virtue of the fact that we live in a modern world with modern luxuries and modern conveniences, most of our diets have strayed away from a good, healthy acid-alkaline blood balance, and maybe some of us without even knowing it is may be living with a chronic condition that results from such a diet known as 'chronic low-grade metabolic acidosis'.

This is what happens when our diet leans to the slightly acidic side for an extended, if not an indefinite amount of time. And the reality is that unless we take active steps to counteract this condition, it is highly likely that we will all succumb to it eventually, if not already. That is just the nature of the world we live in and the habits and practices of the industries and populations of our societies.

So if you are suffering from a form of low-grade chronic metabolic acidosis, perhaps without even knowing it, what are the signs? For one thing, you may notice some weight gain. This is a result of inefficient metabolic function on account of long-term low-grade acidosis. You may also suffer from pronounced but unspecific aches and pains. These will often be in the joints or even the bones. This type of pain associated with low-grade acidosis is likely the result of an acid buildup in the joints and bones.

Acid reflux, predictably, is also a good sign of this prevalent condition. But that is not the only part of your digestive system that can be affected. Long-term, low-grade acidosis can also cause a number of other digestive issues like intestinal cramping, irritable bowel, and generally poor digestion.

A whole host of other issues could manifest if you are one of the high percentages of people who unknowingly live day to day with a chronic case of low-level metabolic acidosis. Chronic fatigue and a general feeling of tiredness and muscle weakness may result. As can a number of other issues like skin problems, bone loss, kidney stones, receding gums, and urinary tract problems. So if you find that you have three or more of the many possible symptoms, then at least eighty percent of your caloric intake should be from alkaline-forming foods. The remaining twenty percent can more or less be of your choosing, but you may find high protein food items to be helpful.

A nice, quick and easy way to boost your body's alkalinity is by drinking beverages that are alkalizing. Spring water is one such naturally occurring source of alkalizing water. Also, water with a dash of lemon juice just as mentioned earlier. Green tea or ginger root tea will also have a similarly alkalizing effect.

You'll want to make sure that you are focusing primarily on eating whole foods. So that means vegetables and fruits, as well as root crops like potatoes and turnips. Also nuts and seeds can be an excellent alkalizing source and also a very strong source of protein. Beans are generally a good choice as well, although lentils, in particular, are renowned for their excellent alkalize boost. And when consuming grains, just remember that it is always best to consume whole grains.

Whether you are pursuing an alkaline diet to target a specific issue, or if you just want to have the healthiest body you possibly can, you are going to want to eliminate as much processed and artificial foods as possible. In fact, that goes for everyone, no matter what. Processed and artificial foods are doing anybody any favors, but they will certainly cause your body's blood pH level to lean to the acidic side. Refined sugars and added sugars rank very high up on the list of these types of foods that should be avoided at all cost. And refined white flour isn't doing you any favors either. In fact, some say it can be just as bad as refined sugars.

And while we are on the topic of eliminating things, if you can handle giving up coffee or any other caffeinated beverages, you will be giving yourself a major advantage on the path to a balanced blood pH level.

There are certain foods and nutritional elements that are acid-forming but that our bodies still need to function properly. These are things that we will have to keep a particularly close eye on in order to monitor amounts of intake. This includes essential fats, as well as pasta and other grains. If you are choosing to continue eating meat, then it should also be noted that meat and fish should both be consumed very sparingly and should also be very closely monitored and limited.

Finally, when it comes to dressing up your greens, namely when being consumed as a salad or being cooked, make sure to use high-grade and healthy fats like extra-virgin, cold-pressed olive oil, avocado oil, and coconut oil. All of which bring along tons of health boosts and benefits in addition to their alkaline-forming properties.

Chapter 7: Alkaline Meal Ideas

Now that we are fully informed and equipped to make good nutrition choices in regards to acid-alkaline blood balance, it is now time to put together some meal plans so we can put all of what we have learned into practice. We are going to look at a prime example of everything you might eat in a day to get the most out of your body.

This particular example isn't about limiting calories of eliminating any particular foods or food groups, so if you have any particular calorie counts you need to stay within, or if you are eliminating certain food groups from your diet such as meat or dairy, you may have to adjust accordingly. Just make sure that if you're replacing anything, to replace it with something of a similar acid-alkaline value, and that it serves that same food role as the replaced item. That is to say, replace proteins with proteins, carbs with carbs, et cetera.

And if you are not calorie counting, obviously use your best judgment here but there is no limit to how many alkalizing foods in the fruits and vegetable categories you can eat. Certainly, you should be limiting acidic foods like meats, dairies, grains, and processed foods if for no reason than to keep your acidity levels down, but fruits and vegetables especially the ones that are particularly alkalizing, you can eat to your heart's content.

So with that said, let's take a look at what our alkaline diet morning might look like.

We wake up nice and early in the morning, refreshed and ready to tackle our day because our healthy, alkaline-rich diet is allowing us to get the sleep we need and preventing our bodies from feeling overly fatigued. The first thing we do is get an ice-cold glass of water, squeeze some fresh lemon juice into it and drink the whole thing as fast as we can. As fast as we can without getting a brain freeze that is!

So now we're going to want to have a nice satisfying breakfast. Today, we are going to do a veggie scramble. Sounds great, doesn't it? This breakfast is going to consist of one or two eggs that we are going to scramble up with green onions, spinach or bok choy or any other leafy greens, and then some chopped bell peppers and diced tomatoes. You can even try it as an omelet if you like. Or even an egg-white omelet if you're feeling really healthy.

Or better yet, if you really want to go healthy, why not try that same breakfast, but as a tofu scramble instead of scrambled eggs. It's easy and delicious. Just replace the eggs with a handful of diced, firm tofu. You can season your tofu however you like, but we recommend trying a chili-style seasoning for some nice, tex-mex style breakfast burritos. Wrap optional.

After that amazing breakfast, we're going to have a nice productive and active morning. If we feel the need for a snack before lunch, we'll have maybe a fruit like an apple or a pear, maybe a banana or a handful of nuts or seeds. An ideal choice would be pumpkin seeds or almonds.

If you're anything like us, that already sounds like an amazing and healthy, nutritious day, but we haven't even gotten to lunch yet. So what might we enjoy for our midday meal on this ideal alkaline diet day? Why limit ourselves, let's look at a couple of options.

For one, we could try some lentil soup. This packs a nice alkalizing punch as it is but combine that with some steamed green like broccoli, carrots, onions, or kale, and you've got a powerful meal. Heck, why not steam up a mix of all of those veggies. Try a light olive oil-based salad dressing on the steamed veggies for some extra flavor.

As delicious as that sounds though, we still have another option. If you're still of the animal eating persuasion, you could try a nice big salmon steak, still a far healthier choice that its terrestrial cousin, served with some mixed greens which could include cucumber, carrots, tomatoes, and broccoli, among pretty much any other fresh veggies you would like. Similarly, you can season that with a light vinaigrette of your choice, but we particularly recommend a lemon and dill based one.

After all that amazing nutrition, you must be ready for a snack! Fight off that mid-afternoon slump with a nice alkalizing snack. This one you can keep nice and simple. Try a simple hard-boiled egg, seasoned with sea salt and fresh ground pepper to taste and a garnish of your choice if you're feeling fancy. Or if you're not inclined toward the animal-based foods, try a straightforward but delicious snack consisting of strips of sweet bell peppers, celery, or carrots, or a mix of all is always an option!

Finally, it's time for dinner and this is where you remaining meat eaters are going to have your way. You can have up to four ounces of your favorite meat, whatever that might be, but we highly recommend that if you must have meat, try to stick to something along the lines of fish, chicken, or other types of light poultry. You can serve this with a side of yam or sweet potatoes, baked or prepared in your favorite way and a nice simple garden salad with mixed greens and a light dressing of your choice.

Or for the plant-based folks, you can indulge in some pasta, but try to find or make pasta made from rice or quinoa, or other grains than wheat. Then you can top your pasta with all kinds of delicious veggies like broccoli, zucchini, and garlic. And then garnish with some olive oil and salt and pepper. Now you've had yourself a fresh and healthy food day!

PART 2

Introduction

Acid reflux is one of the most common ailments affecting adults today. This is due to the notion that there are so many contributing factors and catalysts that can spawn its symptoms. As a result, educating oneself on the best ways to care for the symptoms of reflux is paramount for avoiding and overcoming them once they arise.

Evidently, a common refrain for most reflux sufferers is to avoid foods and drinks that are spicy and or fizzy. While these are certainly helpful approaches to take, you are well advised to consider approaches such as increased exercise for maintenance of overall health, avoiding certain exercises altogether if you are already suffering from severe GERD, implementing dietary changes such as limiting coffee intake, cutting back on peppermint and avoiding highly acidic foods.

But acid reflux symptoms are not caused solely by poor dietary choices alone. Indeed, smoking in excess and excess alcohol consumption are also consistent contributing factors that can induce acid reflux symptoms leading to GERD and Barrett's disease. Leveraging the knowledge presented in this book with regard to the specific dietary and lifestyle changes you must implement, along with acquiring a deeper understanding of the particular scientific reasons for acid reflux, will allow for an informed perspective so that your approach to the symptoms presented is equipped with the most up-to-date and effectual information.

When equipped with these strategies and general knowledge concerning acid reflux, you will certainly be at a distinct advantage when you are confronted by the painstaking and, at its most extreme, life-threatening, symptoms of acid reflux.

Chapter 1: Chronic Acid Reflux & Its Serious Health Implications

Acid reflux is the result of abundant backflow of acid for your stomach into the esophagus. Anatomically, when your lower esophageal sphincter (LES) becomes weakened by, among many causal factors, continually consuming a high diet, acid can flow back into your esophagus causing acid reflux. Consequently, there are numerous symptoms that are spawned by acid reflux including, most notoriously, heartburn and indigestion. While high acidity in the gut is common for everybody and is often devoid of serious health concerns if occurring on a minimal basis, serious health concerns can develop if high acidity can persist for a prolonged period of time. If left unattended and without measures of control put in place, in many instances, these health issues will lead to hospitalization or even death.

In the most serious cases, chronic long-term heartburn, known as Gastroesophageal Reflux Disease (GERD), Barett's esophagus and esophageal problems can arise due to uncontrolled and unaddressed chronic acidity. Some of these most serious ailments are the remnants of years of neglecting the symptoms of acid reflux, particularly after big meals. Over time, the backflow of acid from your stomach damages your esophagus causing erosion of the layers lining the walls of the organ. This inflammation often leads to very painful swelling in esophagus called esophagitis and is accompanied by a painful swallowing feeling. In addition, esophageal ulcers are the most common ailment of an inflamed esophagus. In fact, GERD is the main cause of these ulcers in the lining of the esophagus. Moreover, painful swallowing, nausea, chest pain contribute to a lack of sleep which perpetuates many of these symptoms simplify virtue of that fact that your body is not getting the required rest to overcome these symptoms. As soon as these symptoms arise, be sure to consult a doctor too so that you can be prescribed medication to treat the symptoms before they grow into more serious, persistent conditions. Acquiring medial intervention is especially important when dealing with an ulcer; indeed, ulcers are extremely harmful to the lining of your organ and can be incredibly persistent if left unattended and given time to grow.

Even more, if your highly acidic diet remains the same as before the ulcer, this contributing factor will only enhance the growth of your ulcer and some of your other symptoms. Over time, the scarring of the lining within your esophagus will lead to scar tissue build up, thereby narrowing the esophagus altogether. Swallowing food and drinks will be made much more difficult as a result and may require a surgical procedure to expand the esophagus. These narrow areas of your esophagus are called strictures, and will likely lead to dangerous weight loss and or dehydration. Avoiding a procedure through immediate medical treatment of high acidity is clearly the preferred approach; but once these strictures block your esophageal pathways, a surgical procedure will be required.

Another common ailment of high acidity that affects many people is Barret's esophagus. Specifically, around 10%-15 of people who suffer from GERD will begin to also develop this painful condition, which results in dangerous changes in cells due to excess stomach acid. Thankfully, less than 1% of those who suffer from Barret's esophagus will actually develop esophageal cancer. If intervened early enough in the process, doctors are able to remove any of these abnormally developed cells through a procedure known as an endoscopy, whereby doctors will insert a flexible tube accompanied by a small camera into your esophagus. However, those who have GERD are at a, albeit slightly, increased risk of developing esophageal cancer. Even still, be sure to consult a doctor as soon as your symptoms reach a persistently painful level so that proactive measures and treatment can be implemented to quell your pain, and inhibit the growth of cancer cells.

If there is a long history of esophageal cancer in your family, you will be at an increased risk of developing this cancer as well, especially if you attain medical treatment after a prolonged period of time experiencing symptoms of high acidity. If you are aware of having a family history of esophageal cancer, make sure to ask your doctor for a regular endoscopy to find and mitigate the growth of improper cells. Moreover, tooth decay is a very common symptom of excess stomach acid as it wears down the outer layer of your teeth (enamel). As a result, this can lead to excess cavities and weakened teeth. In a recent study, researchers found that over 40% of GERD patients showed significant tooth decay, along with 70% of patients whose reflux had managed to reach the upper esophagus), compared to only 10% of those patients that had no symptoms of reflux. Certainly, reading about the symptoms that accompany stomach acid is disconcerting and worrisome. Nonetheless, being aware of the symptoms and knowing the early signs of their emergence will mitigate the risks of cancer and other chronic ailments like GERD and Barret's esophagus.

So, what can you do about these symptoms and potentially life-altering health concerns if you are experiencing excess stomach acid? Initially, and rather obviously, begin by assessing your diet. If you typically consume large meals, cut down your portions by at least 25%, and avoid eating right before you sleep. The latter is especially important for your digestive track as your body has to work harder to digest food whilst you are asleep and when your body's organs are supposed to be at rest. Also, limit your chocolate and coffee intake. Typically, medical professionals recommend limiting your coffee intake to only 2-3 cups per day at the most. If these levels are exceeded, your body's acidity levels will climb to healthy proportions and heighten your likelihood of acquiring the aforementioned symptoms. In the same way, excess consumption of alcohol and peppermint carry very harmful side-effects. Not mention, smoking is by far the most dangerous to many of your body's organs, especially the esophagus. Taking steps to cut back and eventually quit smoking is strongly recommended to not only avoid esophageal cancer and weakened tooth enamel, but for a bevy of other health-related reasons not directly associated with stomach acidity. When consulting a doctor to address stomach acid symptoms, you will most likely be prescribed an antacid, H2 blocker or a proton pump inhibitor (PPI); all three are available by prescription as well as over the counter.

Where GERD is concerned, there are other major factors that you should look out for. These symptoms are not specific to a particular body type or even certain foods. First, heartburn is, as mentioned, a clear indicator of GERD and is usually an only an occasional issue that is known to affect over 60 million people at least once or twice a month on average. However, for the 20 million individuals who suffer from heartburn on a chronic level through GERD, seemingly unrelated symptoms can inevitably result in numerous other health complications. You are well advised to consult a doctor if you find that you suffer frequent heartburn (two-three times per week regularly).

When you suffer from GERD, acid, food, as well as digestive juices tend to flow back into your esophagus from the pit of your stomach. Over time, this results in esophagitis, thereby leaving the king of the walls of the esophagus extremely vulnerable to additional harm through scarring, tearing and even deterioration. Additionally, while the primary symptom of GERD is heartburn, there are likely to be other symptoms that are far more difficult to diagnose for doctors and patients alike. Notably, doctors refer to a symptom known as, "silent reflux," which includes voice changes, chronic coughing, major and prolonged throat soreness, along with hoarseness. Patients may have a sustained sensation of having a lump in their throatier having the constant urge for having to clear one's throat. Another common symptom of GERD is the effect that stomach acid has on your breathing. Indeed, GERD, for instance, can heighten the extreme effects of asthma and or pneumonia. Whether or not patients have a history of lung problems personally or with regard to their family lineage, GERD can cause difficulty in breathing and persistent shortness of breath. However, treating this particular symptom is especially tricky; according to several recent studies, GERD medication, like PPIs, have been shown to increase pneumonia by directly contributing to the growth of harmful bacteria. Also, researchers have found that many prescribed PPIs suppress coughing that is needed to clear the lungs. As a result, your doctor may be forced to consider the function of your lungs when prescribing PPIs when in the process of treating symptoms associated with acid reflux.

Many people with ulcers from acid reflux tend to spit up blood and or see it in their stool. For a point of clarity, be sure to note that Esophageal ulcers are much different than stomach ulcers as they (stomach) are usually due to bacteria. Blood from esophageal ulcers, however, tend to be red or a darker purple-red color. If you find yourself having such symptoms, be sure to contact your doctor immediately. The immediate response from your doctor will likely be a schedules endoscopy mentioned earlier. In addition, you may also be prescribed acid-blocking or acid-reducing meds can treat these dangerous stomach ulcer.

An overarching common symptom of acid reflux is a lower quality of life. According to a 2004 study from Europe, whereby 6,000 GERD patients reported that their quality of life had been significantly diminished due to problems that are associated with drink, food and sleep, along with social and physical limitations. Not to mention, there can be major financial implications from having to buy an abundant amount of medications to treat the myriad symptoms of acid reflux, as well as the possible surgical procedures and endoscopy sessions that may be needed if the symptoms escalate to advanced stages. Moreover, the quality of life for patients of GERD was strikingly similar to heart-attack patients and was even lower, in certain cases, for those patients struggling with diabetes and cancer.

Generally, the healing time-frame for GERD is around 2 to 8 weeks. If allowed to persist without medicinal intervention, symptoms of GERD can inflict a considerable amount of damage. For example, reflux esophagitis (RO) can create visible and painful cracks and breaks in the esophageal mucosa. In order to fully and effectively heal RO, acid suppression for a prolonged period (roughly 3-9 weeks) is required and will likely be the timeframe advised by your doctor. Keep in mind that healing rates will rapidly improve as acid suppression increases.

Chronic stress is also a significant factor in the development, growth and. persistence of acid reflux. Our digestive system, moreover, is intricately associated with our nervous system. When stress presents itself, especially in an overwhelming or uncontrollable manner, our digestive system will then receive a lower amount of blood flow, thus causing various issues. Further, our gut bacteria are implicated in our management of stress at increasing levels, so probiotics are helpful in helping the management of this development.

Chapter 2: The Role of Fibre , Prebiotics And Probiotics

Incorporating key changes into your diet can carry massive benefits with regard to dealing with the many symptoms of acid reflux. Specifically, consuming more fiber is an excellent way to mitigate the harsh symptoms. An important point of clarity is the distinction between dietary fiber, defined as edible but non-digestible carbohydrate-based material, and insoluble fiber. Dietary fiber is mainly available in abundance naturally in many cereals, grains, plants, and vegetables as these all play a major role in gastrointestinal health. Given the importance of fiber, and its positive impact in easing the symptoms of acid reflux, many people on average are dangerously deficient in fiber. This deficiency includes both the soluble and insoluble forms of fiber. The main difference between these two forms of fiber are found in their role in digestion; insoluble fiber expedites the travel of foods through the gastrointestinal tract, while solute fibers have been shown to slow the digestion process.

While the varied and, at times, monotonous science concerning acid reflux is still in progress and remains to be settled. Nevertheless, the theoretical benefits of adequate intake of fiber include avoiding trigger foods altogether, as well as the stomach-filling "full" effect of fiber and fewer relaxation reactions of the anti-reflux valve residing between the stomach and the esophagus. Even still, there exists a persistent relationship between acid reflux trigger and the role of fiber. To elaborate, soluble fiber has been shown to induce the body to draw fluid out of already digested food, which then contributes added bulk to your meals which leaves you with a feeling of being "full" for a far more prolonged period of time. As it is commonly found within such sources as barley, peas as well as oat bran, soluble fiber does play an active role in regulating glucose levels and may even contribute to signaling the brain that the stomach is in fact full both during and after eating a meal of any size. Moreover, smaller meals can help acid reflux by refraining from overfilling your stomach. Whereas, insoluble fiber as found within vegetables and whole grains can speed up the passage of stomach contents to your intestinal tract, thereby decreasing your body's propensity for reflux.

Additionally, fatty, fried foods are typically much lower in fiber and are also frequently accompanied by the triggering symptoms of regurgitation, indigestion, and heartburn. Indeed, a fiber-rich diet like fresh fruits, vegetables, and whole-grain bread can tend to contribute to fewer instances of reflux symptoms arising. Some dietary fibers are also widely considered to be probiotics. Note the key distinction between prebiotics and probiotics: the latter refers to the specific helpful bacteria itself, with prebiotic referring to bacterial nutrients. In other words, prebiotics are nutrients which are left for bacteria to digest, or, more plainly, fuel to encourage the balanced bacterial growth within digestive organs. Here, the role of fiber in greatly improving the many symptoms of acid reflux is illuminated; this role is as a bacterial intermediary. On the whole, nonetheless, particular items in your diet tend to perform a seemingly minor role in the symptoms associated with acid reflux. Those who suffer from chronic acid reflux are strongly advised to avoid those specific foods that can aggravate painful heartburn and regurgitation; however, eliminating a broad range of food from your diet is no recommenced as it can detrimental to your overall health. Instead, you should note foods and beverages that can trigger acid reflux specifically and root them out from your diet as soon as possible.

There is a tremendous amount of evidence in favor of incorporating a fiber-rich diet into your daily routine. Notably, the benefits are particular to the overall maintenance of your gut and with regard to managing the amount of harmful bacteria native to that region of your body. A study from 2004 that involved over 65,000 people revealed that fiber intake was associated with the improved perception of acid reflux symptoms. Also, this study revealed people who consumed high fiber bread were nearly three times as likely to experience relief of acid reflux symptoms compared to people who consumed bread with lower fiber content. Granted, the reasons for these results remains unknown; however, the authors of the broad study have speculated that the digestive process of fiber can also be a catalyst for enhanced muscle relaxation from the stomach through the esophagus as it tightens the anti-reflux valve.

So, what are the disadvantages of fiber in acid reflux? It is true that fiber is especially helpful when serving to ease acid reflux symptoms, excess fiber consumption has been shown to aggravate the symptoms. A study published in a medical journalism 2014 indicated that consuming a minimum of 10 grams of highly fermentable starches each day can significantly contribute to painful episodes of acid reflux symptoms. An additional study noted that nine participants who were diagnosed with GERD, those patients who consumed a prebiotic known as fructooligo also had elevated instances of acid reflux symptoms than those patients who were given a placebo.

There are many aspects to consider when striving to efficiently manage acid reflux symptoms. Among them, dietary fiber is perhaps the most important or, at the very least, the most consequential. For instance, while being excessively overweight is certainly risk factor as far as GERD is concerned, adequate consumption of healthy fiber will aid in keeping the weight at a healthy level. Excess fiber, however, causes stomach distension in may people, along with enhanced stomach pressure as well as prolonged emptying on the stomach in many cases, all of which have shown to lead to accentuated acid reflux symptoms. Medical professionals specializing in gastroenterology strongly recommend implementing lifestyle changes such as eating smaller sized meals on a frequent basis (as opposed to larger meals a few times per day), limiting overall consumption of carbonated beverages and foods high in salt content with the intent of improving the acid reflux symptoms. Note that women over the age of 50 should try to consume 25 grams per day; on the other hand, men under 50 are strongly advised to consume 38 grams of fiber each day. While consuming more laxatives is often the approach undertaken by people dealing with symptoms of acid reflux, medical professionals advise increasing your fiber content within your diet for maximized results, as well as maintaining your overall health as laxatives can take a substantial toll on your body and its digestive tract. Consuming a higher amount of fiber will strengthen your stool, keep wastes traveling more smoothly through your intestinal tract, along with preventing constipation. During this process of consuming more fibre, be sure to also ensure that you are consuming plenty of water as well; for fiber to have its absolute best effect, it is imperative that your body remain as hydrated as possible to make sure that waste moves smoothly along your intestinal tract rather than building up due to rigidity.

A good source of probiotics and fiber is yogurt, which carries "good" bacteria helpful for overall maintenance of gut health. A healthy gut is paramount for an efficient and well-functioning intestinal tract and digestive system. Prebiotics and probiotics are, essentially, analogous to food for the bacteria in your stomach; bananas, corn, and whole wheat are additional food sources that are high in prebiotics. Moreover, one of the most beneficial aspects of a fiber-rich diet is the notion that high-fiber foods help control your cravings for snacks. Certainly, high fiber diets can help you lose weight as it displaces other calories for overall maintenance of health.

Guarding against illness, fiber-rich diets will also lower your chances of developing major gut-related illnesses such as diverticulitis. This condition, pockets in the walls of colon trap waste as opposed to moving it along. While doctors remain unsure of the direct catalyst(s) for the illness, consuming a high-fiber diet moves waste fervently along through your system. Along with diverticulitis, a high-fiber diet also eases and prevents irritable bowel syndrome— which has also been linked to acid reflux, albeit a rarer, more extreme symptom. Nevertheless, the most common symptom of acid reflux— heartburn— is quelled by a fiber-rich diet.

Probiotics are becoming increasingly linked to the management of the symptoms associated with acid reflux and alleviating these issues. For a more technical explanation, as we are already aware that probiotics are an effective way of balancing the gut bacteria inside of our bodies, they also help combat against a bacterial infection knows as, H. pylori. This bacterial infection usually originates in childhood. This bacteria, found in the stomach, can alter the environment around them through reducing the acidity levels so that they can survive for longer periods of time. By penetrating the lining of the stomach, thereby remaining hidden and protected by the mucous membrane so that the body's immune defenses cannot reach them. In addition, these bacteria tend to secrete an enzyme called urease, which converts urea to ammonia. The presence of ammonia in this instance is significant because it reduces the stomach acidity around the specific area where the bacteria is found. Coincidentally, it is this lower stomach acid that is often mistaken— by doctors and patients alike— for acid reflux. Can probiotics help combat H. pylori? Well, many medical researchers believe that probiotics can, in fact, help battle this bacteria in several key ways. For one, probiotics are believed to strengthen the protective barrier against H. pylori by producing antimicrobial substances, along with competing against H. pylori for what is known as adhesion receptors (space on the lining of the stomach). Also, it is believed that probiotics assist in stabilizing the gut's mucosal barrier. Many researchers even argue that the production of relatively large amounts of lactate is another inhibitory factor of H. pylori due to the possibility that it could lower the H. pylori urease. Not to mention, probiotics may also be effective in modifying inflammation levels by interacting with the epithelial cells that are responsible for managing the secretion of inflammatory proteins in the gut.

Depending on the particular cause of your acid reflux, probiotics can be incredibly useful for alleviating the painful symptoms. Probiotics can be taken in conjunction with an antacid without worry of the antacid overtaking the positive benefits of the probiotic. More importantly, your approach should be to uncover the root of your acid reflux and adjust medical intervention accordingly. Of course, you doctor plays a huge role in this process, especially in diagnosing the specific cause of your acid reflux; still, it is your responsibility to seek medical expertise so that you can tackle the root of the symptoms as opposed to addressing the individual symptoms as they arise. Being aware of the triggers in both the food and drinks that you consume, managing your stress levels regardless of how often they fluctuate, and finding the specific levels of acid within your stomach are critical steps to address the symptoms of acid reflux. More likely than not, the best method of dealing with your symptoms will be to implement a diverse approach that incorporates a range of approaches rather than relying solely on medical intervention.

Chapter 3: Understanding The Role Of Proteins, Carbs, And Fats In Healing Acid Damage

In recent years, there have been increasing reports concerning the benefits of a low-carb diet in healing the damage induced by acid damage. This may seem counterintuitive given the notion that the standard treatment for GERD includes the *removal* of certain foods that increase acidity in the stomach, for example, tomato sauces which are believed to be contributing causes of excess stomach acidity. Also, as mentioned in chapter 1, the removal of coffee, alcohol, smoking, and peppermint are other dietary and lifestyle changes that ease GERD symptoms. Additionally, researchers have found that diets with a higher amount of carbohydrates can significantly elevate symptoms of acid reflux. Whereas, a low-carb diet has also been shown to reduce symptoms of GERD. While many health researchers and medical experts have expressed concern over the exceptionally low proportion of daily calories from fat and protein in low-carb diets, as wells calorie levels being considerably lower in these diet than recommended. Nevertheless, the effects of gastroesophageal reflux disease have been shown to be significantly reduced after implementation of a low-carb diet. For a case in point, following a 2001 research study in which 5 individuals with diverse ranges of GERD symptoms and across the age spectrum, engaged in a low-carb diet, each of the 5 research participants showed significant relief of symptoms. Granted, throughout the duration of the study, which spanned 8 months, 3 of the 5 research participants also reduced their coffee intake concurrently.

The concurrent reduction of coffee, coupled with lower intake of carbohydrates, was shown to be effective in reducing symptoms such as heartburn and stomach pain. Interestingly, while coffee reduction was a contributing factor, observations from a few of the participants revealed that exacerbating foods such as coffee and fat are less pertinent when a low-carb diet is strictly followed. In other words, when implementing a low-carb diet, the effects of classic factors like coffee and fat intake are vastly diminished even if their consumption is not significantly reduced. So, whether or not you choose to reduce coffee and fat intake significantly, you are likely to reduce most GERD symptoms by solely undertaking a low-carb diet. Therefore, the logical conclusion to draw from these findings is that a low-carb diet is a significant factor for reducing the symptoms of acid reflux. This conclusion gains even more credibility when considering the propensity for high-carb diets to aggravate GERD symptoms.

In addition to lower carbohydrates, lean sources of protein and healthy fats are beneficial for reducing symptoms associated with acid reflux. Lean proteins found in eggs are a great addition to your diet for reducing acid reflux symptoms; however, they are a problem for many people due to elevated cholesterol. If eggs are an issue for you, be sure to consume only egg whites and refrain for consuming higher fat yolks—which have been shown to elevate GERD symptoms. Moreover, as high-fat meals and fried food typically descries LES pressure thereby delaying emptying of the stomach and boosting the risk of acid reflux, it is in your best interest to choose lean grilled meats, as well as poached, baked or broiled meats. Boosting proteins, in the way, will also provide benefits for your overall health as well. Also, complex carbohydrates, as found in rice, whole grain bread, couscous and oatmeal carry excellent benefits for reducing GERD symptoms and easing any scarring that may already be present in the walls of your esophagus. Specifically, brown rice and whole grains add valuable fiber your diet. Root vegetables such as potatoes are excellent sources of healthy carbohydrates and easily digestible fiber. Remember to refrain from incorporating too much garlic and onion while preparing your meals, which are can commonly irritate the esophagus and stomach lining. Along with proteins and complex carbs, incorporating healthy fats has great benefits for easing GERD symptoms and other symptoms accompanying acid reflux. A type of nutrient, fat is high in calories but certainly a necessary component of your diet. Keep in mind, however, fats can vary and they do not all have the same effect on your body. On the whole, you are well advised to avoid consuming a high amount of saturated fats as typically found in dairy and meat, along with trans fats found in processed foods, shortening and margarine. As a replacement, unsaturated fats from fish and or plants are recommended; some examples of monounsaturated fats include sesame, olive, canola, sunflower, peanuts, seeds and nuts, as well as butter. In addition, examples of polyunsaturated fats include such oils as safflower, corn, flaxseed and walnut, fatty fish such as salmon and trout, along with soybean.

Some other helpful tips for reducing acid reflux symptoms include chewing gum, as long as it is not spearmint- or peppermint-flavored. Chewing gum increases the amount of saliva production in your mouth and also reduces the amount of acid in your esophagus. While alcohol consumption has already been mentioned in earlier chapters, research suggests that some people begin to experience extreme symptoms after only one drink; if you fall into this category, be sure to experiment with your levels to uncover what amount is best for you. Additionally, during and after each meal, particularly bigger meals, be sure to remain aware of your posture. Generally, it is a good idea to sit up while you are eating and avoid lying flat on your back for at least hours post-meal. Standing up and walking around the room after a big meal can help encourage the flow of gastric juices in the right direction. Further, avoiding eating big meals before bed can help you refrain from overloading your digestive system while you sleep. Digestion increases the overall amount of gastric acid that is present within your stomach. When laying down, LES's ability to inhibit stomach contents from traveling through the esophagus decreases significantly. When operating concurrently, excess stomach acid and remaining in a reclined position for an unexpended period of time create an abundance of acid reflux symptoms. On the whole, consuming a large meal for less than 3 to 4 hours prior to bed is generally not advisable for those suffering from persistent GERD symptoms; however, the timing of these symptoms can certainly vary depending on the individual.

In a 2017 research study on the benefits of healthy dietary changes versus drug intervention, researchers studied the effects of dietary changes to a type of reflux known as laryngopharyngeal reflux or LPR. This reflux is essentially triggered when pepsin, a digestive enzyme from the stomach, reaches the sensitive tissues in the upper section of the digestive tract. Symptoms like throat clearing and hoarseness are common with pepsin in the throat and or upper part of the digestive tract. In the study, the researchers had participants suffering from acid reflux switch to a Mediterranean diet and consuming significantly more water, thereby neutralizing excess acid. In this particular study, participants avoided classic triggers such as coffee, peppermint, alcohol, fatty and spicy foods, chocolate and soda. Another set of participants were given pharmaceutical drugs to ease GERD symptoms.

After a six week timeframe, participants of the study reported a greater percent of declines in their GERD symptoms as those participants that had used drugs to address the symptoms. Granted, the study did not elaborate on the particular ways in which that the diet and increased water consumption eased the symptoms; nonetheless, the Mediterranean diet incorporates eating mostly plant-based fruits and vegetables. In addition, the increased water can mitigate pepsin's acidity levels in the throat. As mentioned, fruits, vegetables and water are great methods of reducing acid reflux and GERD symptoms. With this in mind, the positive benefits experienced by the study's participants is not surprising in the least. Adjusting your diet for GERD does not require removing all of the foods that you typically enjoy eating. Instead, a few simple changes to your diet if more than enough to address the uncomfortable symptoms of GERD. Your aim in addressing the GERD symptoms should be to create a well-rounded, nutrient-based diet that incorporates a variety of foods that include vegetables, fruits, complex carbs, healthy fats and lean sources of protein. Healing acid reflux damage is made significantly easier when starting with dietary changes that add healthy and diverse foods. Coupled with medical intervention (if required), healthy dietary changes can carry great benefits for healing scarring in your esophagus and stomach, as well as symptoms such as heartburn, bloating and even tooth decay.

Chapter 4: Exercise To Reduce Acid Reflux

When GERD symptoms escalate and you are still in the early stages of implementing dietary changes to address acid reflux symptoms, exercise can be a great option for reducing the symptoms. When GERD symptoms begin to arise, high-impact physical activities like running, skipping rope and jumping exercises. If you are overweight or obese, a weight loss of 10% has been shown to reduce GERD symptoms like heartburn, bloating and reflux. A self-reported analysis study of individuals experiencing GERD symptoms fund that those who reduced their Body Mass Index (BMI) by 2 kilograms or 4.4 pounds or more, along with the circumference of their waist by 5cm or more has improved their GERD symptoms significantly. In contrast, there are also certain exercises that can induce reflux by opening the lower esophageal sphincter (LES) during workouts such as heavy lifting, stomach crunches, or other high impact exercises. When the LES opens, stomach acid travels up into the esophagus causing heartburn.

There are some common sense tips concerning exercise for managing GERD symptoms. First, this twice about how much and what you are eating prior to starting your exercise routine. Obviously, less food in your stomach is ideal. If you are too full, you should wait at least 1 to 2 hours before initiating your exercise routine. This will allow for food to pass fro your stomach through to the small intestine. With less food in your stomach while exercising, it is significantly less likely that you will experience the painful and annoying symptoms of acid reflux such as heartburn and bloating. Next, you should choose the food you consume with thought and, in some instances, caution. Generally, you should avoid foods that trigger GERD symptoms (choosing complex carbohydrates is advised). Your stomach does metabolize these foods much faster than others through a process known as gastric emptying. Moreover, diabetics should avoid high fat and high protein foods before exercise due to being more susceptible to experiencing slow gastric emptying. Experts also suggest adjusting your workout if you suffer from frequent GERD symptoms. Starting at a slower pace with workouts that put less strain on your body like controlled walking and controlled weight training in either a sitting or standing position is strongly recommended. Whereas, high impact, high-intensity workouts like running, rowing and cycling and induce acid reflux. Additionally, acrobatic workouts and gymnastics can also disrupt stomach contents. The key is to avoid exercises that jostle the LES and reflux, these are typically positions that put your body in awkward positions like being upside down defying gravity in one way or another.

A great exercise that carries tremendous benefits for improving and relieving acid reflux symptoms and digestion is yoga. One particular study from 2014 found that six months of yoga significantly reduced acid reflux and stomach bloating, along with improved esophagitis. Again, however, try to avoid positions that heighten GERD symptoms. If any of these "lifestyle" changes fail to improve your GERD symptoms during exercise, be sure to consult your doctor about being prescribed medication for acid-suppression. And, of course, engaging in a constant exercise routine is not only very beneficial with regard to improving your GERD symptoms, but also for the maintenance of your overall health.

Chapter 5: How To Live A Reflux Free Life?

As you may have already noticed, acid reflex can be induced by an abundance of factors ranging from diet, bad habits, poor sleep hygiene, and many other factors. Clearly, it isn't just as simple as cutting out bad habits and instilling a series of great dietary and lifestyle changes. But whether you are able to successfully implement these changes or not does not, thankfully, hinge on strict adherence to a stringent diet or eliminating some of your favorite guilty habits. But before you can begin to consider stepping into a reflux-free life, you should be cognizant of the stages of reflux and recovery.

Firstly, almost everyone who suffers from GERD begins with normal LES and little to no reflux. The severity level of GERD, therefore, more than likely correlates to best with the overall degree of damage inflicted upon the sphincter. Note, however, that this is not easy to determine. Normally, the amount of damage to your sphincter correlates with the overall severity of acid reflux symptoms. This severity is most often determined by the volume, frequency, and duration of reflux episodes. In turn, these factors will correlate with GERD symptoms such as regurgitation and heartburn. If you are diagnosed with GERD, your strategy for addressing the symptoms and eventually overcoming them should first be to containment. Unfortunately, damage to your LES caused by GERD cannot be reversed by drugs and is permanent. Nonetheless, many patients of GERD have been able to live with these symptoms and with functionality despite damage to the sphincter. Changing simple lifestyle habits, such as sleeping and eating, can significantly decrease and prevent severe reflux episodes in spite of damage to your sphincter. In Stage 1 of GERD, known as Mild GERD, most adults currently have minimal damage to their LES and tend to experience mild GERD occasionally. Most often, the adults are left with either tolerating occasional heartburn or will have to use over-the-counter acid suppressive medications from the onset of symptoms through its subsequent stages. Typically, when taking drugs to address the symptoms, quality of life for patients is not affected because the medications are very effective in suppressing symptoms. If you choose to take medication to address symptoms, make sure that you are also cleaning up your diet. If you continue to consume trigger foods and beverages, like coffee and certain sauces, for example, the benefits you garner from medication will be minimal and your recovery will be prolonged if not inhibited altogether. Replacing these meals with smaller, leaner meals that do not pose a threat to inducing symptoms of GERD is recommended. This will ease heartburn and lessen the damage to your sphincter.

In stage 2, known as Moderate GERD, symptoms are far more difficult to control and use of prescribed acid-suppressive drugs will be needed. In this stage, reflux is accompanied by symptoms that are far more intense than stage 1. Therefore, medicinal intervention is needed to mitigate the damage and pain caused by these symptoms. Still, many symptoms in this stage can be managed by using acid-suppressive drugs for prolonged periods of time. Keep in mind that over-the-counter medication can provide insufficient relief; whereas, prescription strength medications are needed in order for you to manage GERD symptoms effectively. Additionally, stage 3, or, Severe GERD, can result in a very low quality if life and is generally considered to be an extremely serious problem by medical professionals specializing in GERD. Because prescription grade acid-suppressive drugs and medicinal intervention usually do not control symptoms, regurgitation is frequent. In Stage 3, it is entirely possible that complications associated with erosive GERD are present. Lastly, stage 4, or, reflux-induced esophageal cancer, is quite obviously the most serious stage. The result of numerous years of severe reflux, nearly 16% of all long-term reflux sufferers progress to this extremely advanced stage. Due to the long-term reflux, the esophagus' lining has been heavily damaged, thereby resulting in a high degree of cellular changes. Also, stage 4 is the stage that involves the pre-cancerous condition called Barrett's esophagus and or an even more severe condition called dysplasia. Granted, these conditions are not cancerous. However, they are capable of raising the risk of developing reflux-induced esophageal cancer. Accordingly, at this stage, common GERD symptoms are likely to also be accompanied by a strong burning sensation in the throat, chronic coughing, and persistent hoarseness. A narrowing of the esophagus, or strictures, will also be present in this stage, and can also be characterized by the sensation that food is sticking to your throat. However, this is only a feeling associated with strictures. Notably, this symptom is also caused by esophageal cancer. Keep in mind that stage 4 GERD can only be diagnosed by a medical professional through an endoscopy and from an intrusive biopsy of cells retrieved from the lower esophagus.

A 30-day recovery plan for GERD symptom can be easily broken into weekly steps. In the first week, you will presumably be trying to lean off of the medication that you have been prescribed. A reversion plan of this nature should take into account a variety of approaches that incorporate dietary changes, exercise routines, sleep schedules, and other lifestyle changes. Drinking more tea and water is strongly recommended throughout your 30-day reversion plan, as long as the tea is not peppermint-flavored. Also, in your first week of recovery, be sure to get as much sleep as possible, in conjunction with eating 2 to 3 hours before you sleep. A meal should also be incorporated throughout this entire 30-day stretch. This plan should include egg whites in the morning, instead of coffee switch to tea for your caffeine fix. For lunch, whole grain bread with lean meat- chicken or turkey preferably- with light sauce and a bevy of vegetables. Moreover, dinner should include a balanced meal that provides nutrients and foods that will not induce heartburn. Remember, this meal should be consumed a few hours before bed so that your body has time to properly digest the food. Also, be sure to refrain from lying directly on your back after your meal; as mentioned, this will induce acid reflux symptoms like heartburn and excess bloating.

In week 2, in keeping with the consumption of nutrient-rich food and water consumption from the previous week, you should begin an exercise routine of you have been devoid of routine prior to week 2. A consistent exercise routine will help maintain overall health so that your body has excess strength and energy to overcome the wear and damage inflicted from GERD symptoms. Also, a consistent exercise routine will boost your metabolism so that you can burn off excess unhealthy fats and complex carbohydrates that can cause strain to your body and induce reflux symptoms. In the third week of your 30-day revision plan, you can slightly increase the size of your meals. Still, make sure that the overall size of your meals remain relatively small, with only slight additions where you may see fit. By week three, your exercise routine, water consumption, and sleep habits should be starting to feel more routine and many of reflux your symptoms will begin to diminish. Moreover, leading into week 4, your diet should continue to incorporate nuts, vegetables, fruits, tea, and other plant-based foods and drinks to expedite the healing process. However, the final week of your 30-day recovery plan is vital for sustaining the progress that you have presumably made since the start of the month. It is vital because you must ensure that you do not get too comfortable in your routine that you allow for gradual decline back into the habits that spawned your acid reflux. Pushing through this final week will augment your progress and solidify your path to living a reflux-free life. Specifically, with regard to your diet, you can incorporate the following fruit and vegetable smoothie recipe. Smoothies and healthy shakes are an excellent meal replacement option for optimal health and recovery from acid reflux.

Add 2 scoops of frozen berries into a 400ml cup

Add 2 scoops of spinach from a 250ml scoop

Add 2 tablespoons of Chia Seeds

Add 2 tablespoons of hemp hearts

Add 1 tablespoon of peanut butter

This smoothie should be blended with water to ensure that it is not excessively thick.

PART 3

Chapter 1: Is Weight Loss Surgery Right for You?

Gastric sleeve surgeries are some of the most life-changing medical procedures a person can go through. The results are often dramatic weight loss and a decrease in health risks. Of course, this type of surgery is a better choice for some people than it is for others. How do you know if you could be a potential candidate for weight loss surgery? The rest of this chapter will provide details about whether bariatric weight loss surgery may be a good option for you.

Guidelines

In order to be considered as a candidate for gastric bypass surgeries, you generally need to have already exhausted other methods for losing weight. Your doctor will most likely ask you about your typical diet, as well as diets and exercises that you have tried in the past. He or she will also need information about your current exercise routine. Your general health and risks of obesity-related health issues will be taken into account as well. In most cases, your BMI (body mass index) must be at least 40 in order to be a candidate for surgery. Sometimes, people who have a BMI of at least 35 are considered. Typically, with the lower BMI of 35, you also have obesity-related severe medical issues such as type 2 diabetes or persistent high blood pressure.

In addition to these guidelines, you will go through the screening processes to determine if weight loss surgery is the best option for you as an individual. The medical team wants to be sure that the surgery will be beneficial to you and that the risks are outweighed by the benefits. Other factors that the medical team will look at are your psychiatric profile, your age, and the level of motivation that you show to become a healthier person with the assistance of bariatric surgery. Surgeries can be performed on teenagers if the benefits greatly outweigh the risks. Bariatric surgeries have also been performed on people who are aged 60 years and over if the benefits are greater than the risks associated with surgery and anesthesia. Prior to surgery, you may be required to show proof that you have made changes to your lifestyle in terms of diet and exercise in preparation for life after your gastric sleeve surgery.

Are you ready for surgery?

Aside from the medical perspective on things, you will have many other questions to ask yourself before deciding if you are ready to go through with a life-altering surgical procedure. You will need to determine how to pay for the procedure. If you have health insurance, you must first receive a pre-approval in order to know what will be covered by the insurance company, and what, if any, portion of the expenses you will be required to cover.

You also have to understand that the surgery itself is not a magical solution. It is only one of the many tools you will use to reach your goal of a healthier lifestyle at a lower weight. In order to reach your full potential after surgery, you will need to be dedicated to a healthier lifestyle. You will have to make nutritional changes to your diet, and you have to start exercising regularly or increase exercise if you are already active. There is also a high probability that you will need to take multivitamins and other supplements, as bariatric surgeries inhibit your body's ability to absorb nutrients.

There are some other points to consider when questioning bariatric surgery for weight loss. People who have struggled with alcohol or medicinal addiction in the past may not be good candidates for gastric bypass surgeries. Similarly, cigarette smokers will need to quit smoking many months before surgery. You will be required to enroll in educational classes before your surgery. Some of these classes will be for you to learn about proper nutrition. This means that you must be able to make time to attend the classes. Some of the screenings that you go through prior to scheduling a surgery may include imaging studies that will monitor your digestive system, as well as blood tests.

Risks associated with surgery

All surgeries have risks that are associated with them that may occur during or after surgery. Weight loss surgeries are no different, and your medical team will help you to measure the benefits and the risks. You will most likely have low levels of calcium, iron, vitamins, and minerals after surgery. This issue can be easily prevented or solved by the addition of daily multivitamins and other necessary supplements. You may experience something called dumping syndrome, which has symptoms of nausea, vomiting, diarrhea, and abdominal cramping. Your intestines may narrow in the areas in which surgery was performed. These narrowed areas are called strictures. If you do not follow recommendations, you may not lose weight or may gain weight back after it is lost. You may also develop a need for another related surgery. Speaking with your doctor will help you determine if you may be a good candidate and if the timing is right for you to undergo a surgery.

Key Points

- Weight loss surgeries are life-changing procedures.

- Surgery in and of itself is not a solution. It is merely a tool that you use in attaining weight loss and a healthier lifestyle.

- You will need to change your eating habits and exercise habits to benefit from surgery.

- You must go through the screening processes to determine if you are a good candidate and which type of surgery will be most beneficial to you.

- The screening processes may include blood testing and imaging sessions.

- You should also consider the financial aspects of surgery, as it can be quite expensive and may or may not be covered by health insurance.

- You will be required to attend educational sessions prior to your surgery to learn about proper nutrition, among other learning opportunities.

- There are risks associated with bariatric surgeries, as with all surgeries. Your doctor will help you determine if the benefits are greater than the associated risks.

Chapter 2: Types of Gastric Sleeve Surgeries

There are four types of gastric bypass surgeries that are among the most commonly performed for weight loss purposes. Each of these kinds of surgeries has associated positive and negative components. There are similarities and differences between the various surgery choices. The four types will be explained below.

It is important to remember that all types of gastric bypass surgery will require changes in diet and exercise in order to reduce health risks and to be successful. You may need to begin taking a daily multivitamin or other supplements due to nutrient absorption issues. You will have the best and healthiest results by working closely with your doctor or surgeon to decide which surgery is right for you, and what your postoperative lifestyle should be like.

Sleeve Gastrectomy

Sleeve gastrectomy limits the size of the stomach by removing a part of it laparoscopically. It works by affecting the amount of food that can be consumed. As a result of the surgery, the hormones are also affected and will assist in the process of losing weight. A benefit is that the hormonal changes can also trigger changes in blood pressure, which will help prevent heart disease. Approximately 80 percent of the stomach is cut away during the surgery, and the organ is left in a tubular shape. The new functional stomach is much smaller than before surgery. Since this is the case, much smaller food portions will be eaten, reducing the overall caloric intake. This option is typically available for people who have a BMI (body mass index) of at least 40. Having this surgery can help you to lose weight and reduce your risk of life-threatening health issues caused by obesity. (Mayo Clinic, n.d.)

Duodenal Switch with Biliopancreatic Diversion

This surgery has two parts. The first part is similar to a sleeve gastrectomy, which removes approximately 80 percent of the stomach. The difference in this surgery is that the pyloric valve that releases food from the stomach is not removed, nor is the duodenum. These two parts will remain in the body. The duodenum is the part of the intestines to which the stomach connects. The second part of this surgery connects the end portion of the intestines to the duodenum. This will cause a reduction in the amount of food that you can consume. It also causes a reduction in the number of nutrients that can be absorbed by the body.

As with sleeve gastrectomy, the new stomach is much smaller, this causes smaller portions to be ingested. The use of less of the intestines contributes to weight loss by reducing the overall absorption of nutrients. The majority of nutrients pass through the digestive system before they are effectively absorbed. This type of surgery is less common than sleeve gastrectomy. It is reserved for people with a BMI of at least 50. The surgery can only be an option if you have already unsuccessfully tried diet and exercise changes to attempt weight loss. It will help you to lose weight and lessen your risk of obesity-related health concerns. (Mayo Clinic, n.d.)

Laparoscopic Adjustable Gastric Banding

The stomach's top section is wrapped around in an adjustable band in this type of surgery. Only a small pouch of the former stomach will remain functional, allowing you to eat less and lose weight. There will be a port placed under your abdominal skin that will allow for the band to adjust. Adjustments are made to the fluid content of a balloon that has been placed under the band. Your doctor can make these changes at appointments, by inserting a needle into the port to add or decrease the amount of fluid that the balloon holds. As with the prior two surgeries, this one also is effective because the functioning amount of the stomach is much smaller. The biggest difference is that the amount of stomach that is portioned off can be adjusted after the surgery is complete. This choice is best for people with a BMI between 40 and 50. If your BMI is over 50, you may not lose as much weight as you desire with this option. (John Hopkins Medicine Health Library, n.d.)

Roux-En-Y Gastric Bypass

This is somewhat the same with the gastric banding but does not specifically use a sleeve or band. It is included here for comparison purposes because it is a common type of bariatric surgery and it also ultimately reduces the size of the stomach. The upper portion of the stomach is stapled off. The result is a pouch that is the size of a chicken egg. The new pouch is attached directly to the intestines, creating a "y" shape. This surgery will help you lose weight by reducing the number of calories and fat that you absorb from foods, along with a reduction in the absorption of minerals and vitamins. After having this surgery, you will be on a modified diet. It will be approximately one-month post surgery before you are able to return to eating normal foods. This option is best for people with a BMI of at least 40. (John Hopkins Medicine Health Library, n.d.)

Key Points

- All gastric sleeve surgeries have risks and benefits associated with them.
- There are similarities that are common factors in the surgeries that are offered, but each surgery has its own sets of positive and negative aspects.
- Most gastric bypass surgeries are performed laparoscopically.
- The duodenal switch with biliopancreatic diversion is ideal for people with a BMI of at least 50. The rest of the commonly performed gastric banding surgeries are ideal for those with a BMI of at least 40.
- Roux-en-Y gastric bypass surgery and duodenal switch with biliopancreatic diversion surgery reduce the absorption of nutrients.
- Laparoscopic adjustable gastric banding allows for adjustments to stomach size to be made by your doctor. You will also be left with a port after surgery so that the adjustments can be completed.
- Discussion with your doctor will help you to determine which surgical choice is best for you.

Chapter 3: The Recovery Phase

Following gastric sleeve surgery, your life will likely look much different than before you started your process as a candidate for the procedure. You will have to take especially good care of yourself and attend all post-op appointments. You will also learn to eat nutritiously with a smaller stomach and developing new exercise routines.

Post-Operative Care

You may spend the first one or two days after surgery in the hospital. This is an excellent time to review any question you might have with your doctor. You might want to go over things such as pain medications, returning to your normal activities, and care for your surgical incision.

You should let your doctor know immediately if you experience any symptoms that could be a result of your surgery. These include a fever, difficulty in breathing, abdominal pain, vomiting, diarrhea, or an incision that feels hot or painful. These could also be signs of infection.

For the first couple of weeks following surgery, you will probably only be permitted to consume a liquid diet. Once you begin to eat regular foods, you must remember to eat slowly while chewing your food well. You will also need to refrain from drinking for a half hour before you eat and for one-half hour after eating.

Nutritional absorption issues may develop after a bariatric surgery. Your doctor will help you to prevent this by telling you to take multivitamins and supplements each day. In addition to a general multivitamin, you may be advised to also take calcium and iron supplements, as well as vitamins D and B12. For the rest of your life, you will most likely take blood tests twice yearly to ascertain your nutritional levels and to determine if any changes should be made to the supplements that you take.

Foods That Promote Recovery and Healing

Some foods are healthier choices than others. After undergoing a weight loss procedure, it is very important to opt for nutrient dense foods that will meet the needs of your diet. There are some foods that are especially noted for their restorative and healing properties such as foods that are high in antioxidants and vitamins. Foods that are rich in vitamins A, C, and D are especially beneficial in aiding healing after surgery. Foods with high levels of vitamin A include dark green vegetables like kale and spinach and orange vegetables like sweet potatoes and carrots. Berries, oranges, melons, tomatoes, and bell peppers are all vitamin C rich. Vitamin D can be found in fish, eggs, milk, and some cereals. Grapes, pomegranates, and all types of berries are full of antioxidants. Antioxidant repair damage to the body. Healthy fats such as nuts, avocado, and olive oil can help your body absorb the vitamins it needs to heal properly. Other highly nutritious foods to ensure you are eating include bok choy, seafood, eggs, beans, and whole grains. Bok choy can contribute to your vitamin K intake, seafood and eggs deliver protein, and beans and whole grains will keep your energy levels up. Yogurt will provide healthy probiotics that will help you with digestion.

Getting In and Staying In Shape with Exercise

Getting proper nutrition is only half the battle in gaining a new healthier lifestyle after weight loss surgery. You will also need to determine what types of exercise will benefit you most and develop a workout routine. You will likely combine some sort of cardio and weight training activities. Always discuss with your medical team to ascertain a safe time to begin adding workouts to your schedule.

Swimming, cycling, and walking are generally the best places to start for low-intensity cardio or aerobic exercises. You will slowly increase your daily activity to add in a stroll through the park, or using the stairs instead of an elevator. Once you get started, you will have an eventual goal of 60 minutes of moderate exercise. Low-intensity exercise is best for weight loss. You will want to exercise on most days, but it is important to take approximately one day a week off to allow your body to rest and make any needed repairs. If you ever feel joint pain, that is not a typical result, and you should make alterations to your exercising routine. The majority of exercise that you do should be of the cardio or aerobic variety, but it is good to add in about 15 minutes of weight training or strength training as well.

Weight training or strength training is fine to add to your workouts up to three times each week. However, you will want to make sure that you space the sessions out by a minimum of 48 hours. Start off slow with light weights and build up as you progress. It is better to have more repetitions than heavier weights to reach a weight loss goal. Lastly, make sure that you are switching up your workouts every six weeks or so. Your body can become complacent with the same exercise routine for long periods of time, so changes are needed to keep your weight loss going.

Key Points

- After your surgery, you will most likely have a short hospital stay.
- Consult with your doctor for the answers to any questions that you may have.
- Be on the lookout for any symptoms of infection.
- Difficulty in the absorption of nutrients is a known side effect of bariatric procedures.
- Nutritional supplements and multivitamins can help to offset difficulty in absorbing needed nutrients.
- Eat small, healthy portions of nutrient dense foods.
- Foods that are rich in protein, antioxidants, and vitamins will be the best for helping you heal after surgery.
- Probiotics are beneficial for digestion.
- Exercise when you have the go-ahead from your doctor.
- Add physical activity slowly.
- Start with light cardio activities and increase exercise until you have six days a week of 60-minute aerobic intervals.
- Adding in weight training or strength training can aid in losing weight and building lean muscle.
- Switch up workout routines often to continue losing weight.

Chapter 4: Recipes for Recovery

While recovering from gastric bypass surgery, you need to be assured that you are receiving adequate nutrients such as vitamins and protein. You will also be eating smaller portions than you are used to after obtaining a gastric sleeve. In order to recover healthfully, it is necessary to eat nutritious foods in variety.

The recipes contained within this book have all been developed especially for patients who have undergone gastric sleeve surgeries. In addition, these recipes contain ingredients that are known to promote healing and recovery and contain nutrition information at the end of each. The serving sizes are all small portions and the foods are delicious. You will find options for breakfasts, lunches, dinners, snacks, and even desserts. Start exploring and choose your favorites!

Egg Muffins

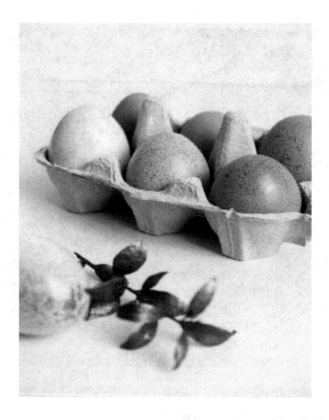

This delicious recipe can be prepped ahead for breakfast on-the-go. Eggs and turkey bacon provide protein to promote healing.

Ingredients:

- Black pepper, .25 teaspoons
- Salt, .25 teaspoons
- 1% milk, .5 c
- Shredded cheese, low fat, .75 c
- Turkey bacon, precooked, 12 slices
- Eggs, 6 large

Preparation Method:

1. Set your oven to 350 degrees.
2. Put one crumbled bacon slice at the bottom of one of the muffin cups of a muffin tin.
3. Except for the cheese, mix all of the other ingredients together.
4. Put .25 c of the mixture in each muffin cup.
5. Sprinkle the shredded cheese over the tops of the muffins.
6. Bake the egg muffins for 20 to 25 minutes.

Number of servings: 12

Size of serving: 1 muffin

- 98 calories
- 7 grams fat
- 2 grams saturated fat
- 1 gram carbohydrates
- 0 gram fiber
- 1 gram sugar
- 8 grams protein

Breakfast Berry Wrap

Berries provide antioxidants needed for healing and whole grains for energy. This breakfast can be prepared quickly and easily, no baking required.

Ingredients:

- Sliced strawberries, fresh, .25 c
- Strawberry jelly, low sugar, 1 Tablespoon
- Ricotta cheese, 3 Tablespoons
- Whole wheat tortilla, 1

Preparation Method:

1. Spread the jelly and the ricotta cheese on the tortilla.
2. Sprinkle the strawberries.
3. Roll the tortilla up and serve.

Serving size: 1 wrap

Number of servings: 1

- 229 milligrams sodium
- 233 calories
- 24 milligrams cholesterol
- 30 grams carbohydrates
- 9 grams fat
- 8 grams sugar
- 8 grams protein

Black Bean and Corn Salad

A delightful mixture of beans and corn will provide protein and energy. There is no cooking necessary, so this recipe is easy enough for anyone to try out.

Ingredients:

- Whole kernel corn, 1 cup
- Lemon juice, 1 teaspoon
- Minced garlic, 1 teaspoon
- Olive oil, 2 Tablespoons
- Honey, 1 teaspoon
- Black pepper, .25 teaspoons
- Minced red onion, 2 Tablespoons
- Balsamic vinegar, .25 cups
- Drained and rinsed black beans, (2) 16 oz cans
- Fresh parsley, .25 cups

Preparation Method:

1. Mix the corn, black beans, red onion, and pepper in a large mixing dish.
2. All of the other ingredients should be whisked.
3. Pour the liquids over the mixture.
4. Marinate the salad for 30 minutes before serving.

Serving size: .25 c

Number of servings: 6

- 306 milligrams potassium
- 40 milligrams sodium
- 0 milligram cholesterol
- 6 grams protein
- 3 grams sugar
- 6 grams fiber
- 23 grams g carbohydrates
- 5 grams fat
- 160 calories

Baked Chicken and Vegetables

A classic dinner takes on a new life in this recipe. Cook dinner for the family or meal prep and have this recipe for lunches and dinners. Protein and vitamin A will aid in the recovery.

Ingredients:

- Black pepper, .25 t
- Thyme, 1 teaspoon
- Water, .5 c
- Raw skinless chicken, 1
- Quartered onion, 1 large
- Sliced carrots, 6
- Sliced potatoes, 4

Preparation Method:

1. Preheat your oven to 400 degrees.
2. Put the carrots, potatoes, and onions in a large oven-safe dish.
3. Place the chicken over the vegetables.
4. Mix up the water, black pepper, and thyme.
5. Pour this mixture over the vegetables and chicken.
6. Spoon the cooking juices over the chicken two times while cooking. Bake for at least one hour until the chicken is browned.

Serving size: one-sixth of the recipe

Number of servings: 6

- 130 milligram sodium
- 26 grams protein
- 10 grams sugar
- 4grams fiber
- 25 gram carbohydrates
- gram fat
- 240 calories

Asian Style Lettuce Wraps

Full of flavor, this recipe provides you with plenty of protein! This one is great for a group or as a make-ahead meal.

Ingredients:

- Sliced cucumber, 1 small
- Chopped green onion, 1 whole
- Butter lettuce, 8 leaves
- Sesame oil, toasted, 1 teaspoon
- Minced ginger, 1 teaspoon
- Ground chicken breast, .5 lb
- Minced onion, 1 c
- Minced garlic, 1 Tablespoon
- Splenda, 2 packets
- Sriracha hot sauce, 2 teaspoon
- Peanut butter, unsalted, 1 Tablespoon

- Soy sauce, low sodium, 2 teaspoons
- Hoisin sauce, 2 Tablespoons

Preparation Method:

1. Combine hoisin sauce, sriracha, peanut butter, soy sauce, and Splenda in a bowl and mix well.
2. Place a nonstick skillet over medium heat.
3. Cook the onion for four minutes. Mix in the garlic and cook for one more minute.
4. Add the ground chicken and ginger.
5. Increase the temperature of the burner to medium-high heat.
6. Break the chicken up and cook it until there is no pink color left.
7. Stir the sesame oil in and remove from the heat.
8. Divide the product evenly among the lettuce leaves.
9. Top with cucumber and green onion.

Serving size: 2 wraps

Number of servings: 4

- 637 milligrams sodium
- 33 milligrams cholesterol
- 16 grams protein
- 4 grams sugar
- 5 grams fiber
- 11 grams carbohydrates
- 4 grams fat
- 155 calories

Cheesesteak Wrap

Yes, you can still enjoy a chicken cheesesteak. With a few tweaks to the original, this recipe contains protein, vitamin C, and antioxidants.

Ingredients:

- Low carb tortilla, 1
- Light Swiss cheese, .75 oz
- Sliced mushrooms, .25 c
- Sliced green peppers, .25 c
- Chopped onions, .25 c
- Skinless, boneless chicken breast, .25 lb

Preparation Method:

1. Pound the chicken breast until it is .25 inch thin. Then create thin strips by cutting it with a knife.
2. Cook the chicken on the medium-high heat in a cooking pan with the onions.
3. Add the mushrooms and the green pepper and continue cooking.
4. Warm the tortilla for 20 seconds in the microwave, then place in the middle of two damp paper towels.
5. Spread the cheese in the middle of the tortilla.
6. Add the vegetables and the chicken.
7. Fold up the tortilla and serve.

Serving size: 1 wrap
Number of servings: 1

- 620 milligrams sodium

- 76 milligrams cholesterol

- 3 grams protein

- 4 grams fiber

- 264 calories

- 17 grams carbohydrates

- 6 grams fat

Beef Ginger Stir Fry

Instead of going out, try to make a stir-fry for you at home. This recipe provides plenty of protein, vitamin A, and whole grains for energy.

Ingredients:

- Water chestnuts, 8 oz
- Bok choy, 2 medium stalks, cut in .5 inch slices
- Brown rice, instant, .5 c
- Medium bell pepper, .5 cut in strips
- Broccoli florets, 3 oz
- Red pepper flakes, crushed, .25 teaspoons
- Soy sauce, 3 Tablespoons
- Cornstarch, 1 Tablespoon
- Canola oil, 1 teaspoon
- Beef broth, 6 oz fat-free
- Garlic cloves, 2 medium
- Ground ginger, 2 teaspoon
- Flank steak, 1 lb (in .25 inch strips)

Preparation Method:

1. Mix the garlic, ginger, and steak slices in a bowl and set it aside.
2. Stir the broth, soy sauce, and cornstarch together in a separate bowl.
3. Heat the oil in a skillet over medium-high heat. Add the pepper flakes.

4. Constantly stir the steak while cooking it for four to five minutes, and then set it aside.

5. Cook the bell pepper and broccoli for two to three minutes. Then add the water chestnuts and the bok choy.

6. In the center of the pan, make a well to put in the broth.

7. Cook this for one to two minutes, and then mix the beef in and cook for an additional one to two minutes.

8. Serve the stir-fry over the rice.

Serving size: .25 of the total

Number of servings: 4

- 17 grams protein
- 6 grams sugar
- 2 grams fiber
- 25 grams carbohydrates
- 8 grams fat
- 275 calories

Zucchini Boats

Chock full of antioxidants and protein, this recipe will assist in healing. It makes many servings, so this is a good recipe for making ahead or for a family dinner.

Ingredients:

- Low-fat shredded mozzarella cheese, 1 c
- Black pepper, .25 t
- Whole wheat bread crumbs, .25 c
- Spaghetti sauce, .75 c
- Diced tomato, 1 large
- Sliced mushrooms, .5 lb
- Beaten egg, 1
- Chopped onion, .5 c
- Ground turkey, 1 lb
- Zucchini, 4 medium

Preparation Method:

1. Slice the zucchinis lengthwise in half. Scoop out the pulp to create boats and set it aside.
2. Put the boats in a large dish safe for use in the microwave. Cover the dish, and then heat it in the microwave for three minutes on high.
3. In a skillet, cook the onion and turkey on the medium-high heat.
4. Drain the turkey mix.

5. Mix the zucchini pulp, egg, bread crumbs, spaghetti sauce, tomato, mushrooms, cheese, pepper, and turkey mix.

6. Place a quarter cup of the mix into each one of the shells.

7. Bake for 20 minutes, uncovered, at 350 degrees.

Serving size: 1 boat

Number of servings: 8

- 294 milligrams sodium
- 17.5 grams protein
- 5 grams sugar
- 4 grams fiber
- 16 grams carbohydrates
- 7.5 grams fat
- 195 calories

Veggie Pizza

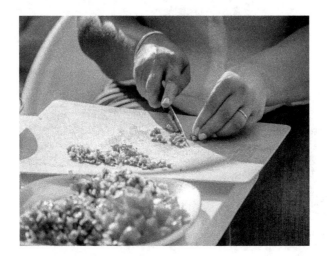

This recipe is fun for parties or an evening at home. Plenty of vegetables make it great for recovery and healing.

Ingredients:

- Black olives, .5 c sliced
- Shredded Colby jack cheese, low fat .75c
- Diced cucumbers, .25 c
- Diced green pepper, .25 c
- Diced tomatoes, .25 c
- Diced broccoli, raw .75 c
- Shredded carrots, .25 c
- Ranch dressing dry mix, 1 package
- Sour cream, low fat, .5 c
- Cream cheese, low fat, .5c
- Large low carb wraps 2

Preparation Method:

1. Mix the ranch dry mix, sour cream, and cream cheese until combined.
2. Spread the ranch combination on the tortillas.
3. Use the vegetables as toppings.
4. Sprinkle the cheese over the top.
5. Divide the tortillas into quarters and serve.

Serving size: .25 tortilla

Number of servings: 8

- 870 milligrams sodium
- 23 milligrams cholesterol
- 10 grams protein
- 1.6 grams sugar
- 4 grams fiber
- 12 grams carbohydrates
- 10 grams fat
- 170 calories

Hummus

This is a classic hummus recipe. Use it for a vegetable dip or for salads.

Ingredients:

- Salt, .5 teaspoon
- Chickpeas, (1) 15 oz can rinsed
- Lemon juice, 3 Tablespoons
- Olive oil, 3 Tablespoons
- Tahini, 1 Tablespoon
- Garlic, clove 1 peeled

Preparation Method:

1. Chop the garlic in a food processor.
2. Add all of the other listed ingredients.
3. Blend the ingredients one to two minutes, until entirely smooth.

Serving size: 2

Number of servings: 12

- 149 milligrams sodium
- 0 milligram cholesterol
- 6 grams protein
- 0 gram sugar
- 72 calories
- 7.5 grams carbohydrates
- 4.5 grams fat

Spicy Devilled Eggs

This is a great snack to have on hand for a little protein. You can make it ahead and have it ready.

Ingredients:

- Paprika a dash
- Black pepper a dash
- Hard boiled eggs, 6 whites, 3 yolks
- Dijon mustard .25 t
- Dill .5 t
- Greek yogurt 2 T

Preparation Method:

4. Peel all of the eggs and slice them lengthwise in half.
5. Set aside the whites. Put three yolks in a bowl to mix.
6. Mash the yolks with the yogurt, dijon, and dill.
7. Spoon the filling in the half eggs.
8. Sprinkle paprika and black pepper on the tops of the eggs.

Serving size: 2 egg halves

Number of servings: 3

- 219 milligrams sodium
- 225 milligrams cholesterol
- 10 grams protein
- 0 gram sugar

- 131 calories
- 1 gram carbohydrates
- 8.7 grams fat

Soy Chocolate Dessert

This is a recipe for a pudding made with tofu. The tofu makes the dessert creamy and healthy, and the protein helps you heal.

Ingredients:

- Vanilla extract, .5 t
- Silken tofu, 16 oz
- Skim milk, 1 c
- Fat-free, sugar-free chocolate fudge pudding, instant, 1 package
- Hot water, .25 c
- Unflavored gelatin, 1 envelope

Preparation Method:

1. Mix the hot water and gelatin in a small bowl and allow it to set.
2. Dice the tofu in one-inch cubes and put it in a mixing bowl with the pudding.
3. Add vanilla extract and place the mixture in a blender.
4. Blend until you reach a smooth texture, and then add the gelatin gradually until well-combined. Blend once more.
5. Pour the mix in an 8-inch by 8-inch dish.
6. Cover and leave the dish in the refrigerator for at least 30 minutes.

Serving size: .5 c

Number of servings: 8

- 181 milligrams sodium

- 1 milligram cholesterol
- 5 grams protein
- 6 grams carbohydrates
- 1 grams fat
- 56 calories

Cheesecake Pudding

Here is a dessert that takes no time at all to make. Greek yogurt provides protein that is needed for the healing process.

Ingredients:

- Cheesecake flavored pudding mix 1 packet, sugar-free
- Greek yogurt 1 c, plain, fat-free

Preparation Method:

1. In a blender, puree the ingredients until they are combined.

Serving size: .5 c

Number of servings: 2

- 7 grams protein
- 4.5 grams sugar
- 3 grams carbohydrates
- 0 grams fat
- 62 calories

PART 4

Introduction

This book has a very wide range of people it can help. Whether you're just considering Bariatric surgery, trying to figure out if you'd be a good candidate, or if you have the date set for surgery and you want to know what to expect and how to prepare, want to know about post-op care and recovery, or how to maintain your body after surgery, this can help anyone from the beginning steps all the way until months after. You'll find out what the requirements are for surgery and if you can qualify, the different kinds of procedures and the pros and cons of each one, how you'll need to prepare and what diet restrictions you'll have after surgery. This book will also include foods that you can and can't eat before and after surgery along with a meal guide for after your procedure. This will be the beginning of a whole new lifestyle for you so congrats on taking the first step to making that change!

Chapter 1: What? Who? And Why?

What is Bariatric surgery? By definition, Bariatric surgery is a surgical procedure performed on the stomach or intestines to induce weight loss. Weight loss is achieved by wrapping a gastric band around the stomach to reduce its size or by re-routing the small intestine to a small stomach pouch. The procedure causes weight loss by restricting the amount of food the stomach can hold. The most common types of procedures are Gastric Bypass, Gastric Sleeve, Adjustable Gastric Band, and Biliopancreatic Diversion with Duodenal Switch (BPD/DS).

- Gastric Bypass
    - This is done by dividing the top part of the stomach, then dividing the first portion of the small intestine and attaching it to the top piece of the divided stomach.
    - Pros: On average you'll lose 60%-80% of your excess weight, restricts the amount of food you can consume, can lead to increased energy, positive changes in gut hormones that enhance satiety and reduce appetite.
    - Cons: It's a more complex operation compared to the other procedures, which could result to more complications, it could lead to long-term vitamin/mineral deficiencies (particularly in Vitamin B12, iron, calcium, and folate), typically a longer hospital stay is required compared to other procedures, requires following your doctor's dietary recommendations, and could lead to life-long vitamin/mineral supplementation.
- Gastric Sleeve

- o This procedure is done by removing 80% of the stomach. The new stomach holds much less than the normal stomach so there's much less calories being consumed.

- o Pros: It restricts the amount of food that your stomach can hold, induces significant weight loss in a short amount of time, and it does not require any foreign objects or rerouting the food stream, normally a short hospital stay (about 2 days), and causes changes in gut hormones that suppress hunger, reduce appetite and improve satiety.

- o Cons: The procedure is non-reversible, there is a possibility of having long-term vitamin/mineral deficiencies, and there is a higher chance of an early complication rate.

- Adjustable Gastric Band

  - o This involves putting an inflatable band around the upper portion of the stomach. This creates a smaller stomach pouch above the band.

  - o Pros: Reduces the amount of food that can go into the stomach, typical weight loss of about 40%-50% of your excess weight, it does not involve any cutting or rerouting, requires a much shorter hospital stay compared to other procedures (usually around 24 hours or you can even be released the same day), this procedure is reversible, has the lowest rate of early post-op complications, and has the lowest risk for vitamin and mineral deficiencies.

  - o Cons: This procedure has the highest rate of re-operation, it requires sticking to a strict post-op diet and going to your post-op follow up visits, dilation in the esophagus can result if you overeat, you may experience mechanical problems with the band, procedure requires a foreign device to remain inside of your body, a higher percentage of patients fail to lose up to 50% of excess body weight, less early weight loss, and slower weight loss compared to other procedures.

- Biliopancreatic Diversion with Duodenal Switch (BPD/DS)
  - There are two parts to this procedure. First, a portion of the stomach is removed, leaving a tube shaped stomach. Then, a large portion of the small intestine is bypassed.
  - Pros: Average weight loss is about 60%-70% of your excess weight at a 5 year follow up which is much greater than other procedures, it is the most effective procedure against diabetes, causes changes in gut hormones that improves satiety and reduces appetite, reduces fat absorption by 70% or more, and it also allows patients to eventually eat more "normal" meals.
  - Cons: There is a higher risk compared to similar procedures, requires a longer hospital stay, requires a very strict compliance with follow up visits and dietary/vitamin supplementation recommendations, and guidelines are critical to avoiding serious complications such as protein and vitamin deficiencies.

If you have been considering Bariatric surgery, I hope the list above has given you some things to consider when you think about which procedure would be right for you. Depending on which procedure you have done that can affect how long you're in the hospital, your recovery time and how much weight you lose after the surgery.

Who would be a good candidate for Bariatric surgery? If you are considering surgery, then there are a few things you need to ask yourself first. One of the first questions you need to ask yourself is what is your BMI? If you have a BMI over 40, then most organizations would say that weight loss surgery is a reasonable option for you, but you must be healthy enough to sustain surgery. To give you an example, if your height is 5'5" then your BMI would be 40 if you weighed 240 ½ pounds. The next question you should ask yourself is do you have any weight related medical conditions? In some cases, certain medical conditions may help qualify you for surgery, but others might make you not able to withstand the procedure. If you have a BMI of 35 or over, you may qualify for surgery if you have at least one obesity related medical condition such as Type 2 Diabetes, hypertension, gastrointestinal disorders, heart disease, non-alcoholic fatty liver disease, osteoarthritis, lipid abnormalities, sleep apnea and other respiratory disorders.

Why should you consider Bariatric surgery? Most people that are considering having these procedures done or already have had them done have tried other weight loss options and have not been successful with them. If it's at all possible to avoid surgery, then you should go with that option since all procedures are not without their own risks. Some examples of a non-surgical option to losing weight would be diet and exercise, a support group or a partner who will motivate you, supplements or weight loss medication. If you haven't tried any of these options, then you may not qualify for surgery.

We now know what Bariatric surgery is and the different procedures that are available. You should pick the procedure that will best fit your needs and consider all the risks that comes along with each procedure, along with the benefits. Some procedures have higher risks than others and some can make you lose a higher amount of weight in a shorter amount of time. You should consider both the risks and benefits when choosing one. Once you've weighed your options and you have figured out if you would be a good candidate and why you want the surgery, that will better help you in finding out which one would be the best option for you. Once you know which procedure you will be doing, we can move on to how you can prepare for you big day.

Chapter 2: Preparing for Surgery

This surgery is a big step into your new lifestyle. In order to prepare you'll have to make a few changes. First, if you are a smoker then it will be required that you stop smoking before your surgery. This will reduce the risk of some complications after surgery. If you don't quit smoking before surgery it can cause breathing problems before and after the procedure, and you'll have a higher risk of developing pneumonia. Smoking also slows down your blood flow, which means you won't heal as fast. On top of that making your recovery time much longer, that also means you are at risk of infection for a much larger period of time than you normally would have been. It's recommended that you quit smoking at least a week in advance. But even quitting just one day in advance can decrease your chances of complications, although the earlier the better. You will also need to stick to any medications your physician has prescribed you along with any dietary restrictions that were given to you. Unless given a diet to follow by your doctor, here is a diet that you should follow at least 3 weeks before your surgery.

- You should be eating at least 60 grams a day of protein.
- Eliminate all refined sugars and reduce carb intake.
- Eat healthy fats, avoid bad kinds of fat.
  - Healthy fats: Avocado, fish, nuts, olives, etc.
  - Bad fats: Butter, vegetable oil, fast food, cake, etc.
- Avoid high calorie foods.
- 48-72 hours before surgery you should be on an all liquid diet. Do not consume any solid food.

- The night before your surgery you should stop consuming all liquids and food. This allows the surgeon to operate without any interference.

You also may need to stop taking certain medication before surgery. Inform your doctor of any medication you are taking so they can tell you what is and isn't safe to be taking before surgery. Medications you may need to stop taking include arthritis medication, NSAIDS (nonsteroidal anti-inflammatory drugs such as Tylenol, Aspirin, Ibuprofen, Naproxen), and any anticoagulants (Enoxaparin, Clopidogrel, Dipyridamole, Ticlopidine, and Warfarin). Any medication that acts as a blood thinner should be removed from your diet to remove the risk of complications during surgery.

Other planning may be needed depending on the length of the hospital stay and your recovery time. These can vary based on which procedure you are having done. You may want a family member, close friend or spouse to stay with you at the hospital or at home with you for support once you are released. It is also a good idea to make home and/or work arrangements since you will be recovering for a few weeks.

You will also need to mentally prepare yourself for surgery and for life after. You need to find the root cause of your weight gain. Is it because of a health issue? Stress? Is it because of depression or a food addiction? Many people who are obese whose cause is not related to a health issue may have problems with food addiction. It is imperative that you know food addictions not dealt with after surgery can have dire consequences. You can severely harm yourself if you continue the food addiction after you have the surgery. The reason this is so important is because when you eat large amounts of food it can cause your stomach to rupture. This can happen with a normal stomach so your chances of having your newly, much smaller stomach rupture rapidly increase. Having this procedure done will not make food addictions go away. That is a lifestyle change that only you can make. You must want to change, surgery or no surgery. If you don't, you will have severe consequences to deal with.

Preparing for your procedure may be a little tough but it's preparing you for your new lifestyle ahead. Since you'll be recovering for a little while after surgery remember to take care of any responsibilities you may have over the next few weeks and to not have anything to eat or drink for the 24 hours leading up to the surgery. It may be hard to do but keep your goals in mind and let them motivate you.

Chapter 3: Your Surgery Day!

After all the time you've spent preparing, it's finally here. It's time to get your surgery! The morning of your procedure there are still a few last preparations. Any medications you are still taking should only be taken with a sip of water, anything that could be lost or is going to be taken off should be left at home, and wear something comfy. You're going to be here for a while, so you should make yourself comfortable. You've been eating a pretty restrictive diet lately and have consumed nothing at all the past 24 hours. On top of that you're probably feeling nervous. Don't freak out, it's completely normal to feel this way but knowing what to expect can help you to relax. When you arrive at the hospital, you'll sign some paperwork and get checked in, then you'll be taken back to an examination room. Here you'll do your pre-op physical, EKG (a process that records electrical activity of the heart) and have some blood/lab work done. Then a physician will come out to go over your procedure and this is when any questions you may have can be asked and answered. You'll be given an I.V. and then you'll wait until someone comes to get you. When they come to get you to bring you back for surgery you will be taken back to the operating room on a stretcher. Your family/friends that are there with you will go wait in the waiting room until you are done with your procedure. Before your surgery starts your anesthesiologist will give you a medication and you'll go to sleep.

A nurse will notify your family when your surgery is complete and the surgeon that performed on you will speak to them in the waiting room Depending on the type of procedure you had done, you'll either wake up on a stretcher or a hospital bed. You will always have an R.N. available to you and if you need any pain medication then there will be a button for you to push. Discomfort after surgery is normal but report if you feel any sudden/severe pain or shortness of breath. Some common complaints are shoulder pain, soreness on the left-side abdominal area, nausea, constipation/diarrhea, gas pain, weakness, and fatigue. Keep in mind this is just a guideline. This is a researched example to give you an idea of what to expect on the day of your surgery.

Congratulations, you made it! I'm sure you're excited and will want to know how much weight you can expect to start losing. You should ask your doctor, but your results can be varied depending on multiple factors. This depends on which procedure you had done, how much you weigh now, and how you take care of yourself from here on out will all contribute to your weight loss results. Most people lose about 60% of their excess weight after gastric bypass surgery. Now that you're done with your surgery and are now recovering, you can learn about post-op care.

Chapter 4: Post-op Care

Before we talk about post-op care, I'm going to include some side effects that you might experience after surgery and include if they are just a common side effect, or if they can seriously harm you so you'll know what to look out for.

- Constipation (common)
    - This is very common after weight loss surgery. Inform your doctor and they will instruct you on what to do.
- Gallstones (common)
    - Up to 50% of patients will develop gallstones after weight loss surgery because it develops when you lose a lot of weight in a short amount of time.
    - 15%-25% of people will need surgery to remove their gallstones after gastric bypass surgery.
    - Gallstones can also cause nausea, vomiting and abdominal pain.
- Blood clots in your lungs (serious)
    - This is rare, happening only 1% of the time but is still a possibility.
    - Although this can be life threatening, blood thinning drugs can usually prevent blood clots. Frequent activity can also prevent it.
- Bleeding in stool (serious)
    - This can appear reddish or black and is very serious. Inform your doctor immediately.

- Dumping Syndrome (common)
  - This can happen if you eat meals that are high in sugar after weight loss surgery.
- Wound infections (common)
  - This can happen up to 3 weeks after surgery.
  - Symptoms include redness and warmth, pus, and pain from the wound.
  - Requires antibiotics and could possibly need surgery.
- Leaks (serious)
  - Rare, but serious.
  - Can occur up to 5 days after surgery.
  - Symptoms include abdominal pain and feeling ill.
  - Call your doctor if you think that you are experiencing this.

Post-op care is very important, especially for weight loss surgery. As previously mentioned, you can severely harm yourself by not following certain guidelines. Dietary guidelines are extremely important to follow, and they are critical to your health, recovery and success with your weight loss journey. Vitamins and minerals are also very important to take because they will give you the nutrients that you need after your surgery. Most procedures also cause vitamin and/or mineral deficiencies so taking them will help to prevent that. It would be a good idea to incorporate some exercise into your routine, daily physical activity is important. It's recommended that you get 30 minutes each day. There are also support groups if you want some extra help to stay motivated. These groups are for people who have had weight loss surgery and would like to share advice, thoughts and concerns, ask questions, and overall give support. If you aren't comfortable with a group maybe you can find a family member or a close friend that is interested in doing this journey with you and you can motivate each other to reach your goals.

Although your surgeon will probably give you a list of recommended foods, some of the food items for a Bariatric surgery post-op diet are tea, sugar-free, non-carbonated beverages, non-acidic juices, broth (chicken, beef, vegetable) cottage cheese, oatmeal, and cream of wheat. There is a diet progression which you MUST follow. This is extremely important, if you try to eat something that is too solid too soon then you could possibly rupture your stomach. The diet progression goes clear liquids, full liquids, pureed foods, soft foods, and then finally solid foods. It could take 4-12 weeks for you to go through the entire progression. How quickly you go through it can depend on the type of surgery you had, speed of recovery, and your body's natural tolerance to the food progression. During the clear liquid diet phase, you can only drink liquids that are see through. This includes tea, water, diluted fruit juice that is non-acidic, protein fruit drinks, sugar-free gelatins, and artificially sweetened non-carbonated drinks. Once your body can handle clear liquids, you can move onto the full liquid phase. In this phase you can have protein shakes, skim milk, low-fat cream soups, low-fat yogurt, sugar-free gelatin, and sugar-free pudding. The next phase is pureed foods. This is soft food blended up to have a smoother consistency, to make it easier for your stomach to handle and does not have any chunks in it. The type of food that is included in this has a pretty large range because it doesn't have to originally be soft since it's getting blended. Next is the soft food phase and this is when you can start eating actual food again, but it needs to be easy to chew. This can include steamed vegetables, soft fruit, pasta, and oatmeal. Even though your eating soft foods it can still be hard on your stomach. Make sure your food is mushy and you've thoroughly chewed it before swallowing. It will probably take you 30-60 minutes to finish a meal if you are chewing properly. I know this may seem tedious, but it's very important that your food is completely chewed so that it is easier to digest. It may tire you now while eating but you'll thank yourself later when your stomach can digest what you've eaten. The last phase is the solid food diet. Once you can normally eat soft foods again you can move onto this phase. You should slowly add solid food to your diet and more and more will be added gradually so that your digestive system can get used to the solid food. You should still be chewing slowly and thoroughly even at this phase. Once again I know it may seem like you can handle it but your stomach is very sensitive right now and even when you move up to solid foods, especially when you move to solid foods, you'll need to chew thoroughly and slowly to take it easy on your stomach. Along with the dietary progression you should be following dietary guidelines as well so that you are getting the nutrition that your body needs. You should choose healthy foods that are low on fat and high in protein. Remember to drink plenty of fluids throughout the day but avoid drinking with meals. One of your biggest concerns is going to be making sure you're eating enough protein. Protein is not something that the body replenishes. For women, the daily requirements are 50-60 grams. For men, the requirements are 60-70 grams. You may need to take protein supplements to meet your daily requirements after surgery.

Something that you'll have to be slow and consistent with is your fitness after surgery. It's important to keep you body healthy and this will help you work towards your goal. After surgery if you are planning on exercising, take it very SLOW. There are countless people that tried to do too much, too soon after their surgery and ended up bedridden for a week or more. This will set you back quite a bit as far as your fitness goals are concerned so if you really want to keep progressing then you will be extra careful to not go too far. In the days immediately following your surgery, the medical team will be telling you to walk as much as you can. You should spend the first few days at home getting up out of bed and walking around the house. Any physical activity is good, get up and walk around if you're bored or to watch T.V. It seems like it's pointless but it's really not. Any kind of exercise will increase the blood flow in your body. By moving around, this tells your brain that your muscles are being used and this will burn calories. The only thing that you are able to consume right now is a protein shake, so you aren't consuming any substantial amount of calories. When your body burns calories and they aren't being replenished then it will have to pull those calories from somewhere and start dipping into your fat reserves, this burns fat! At a few weeks out form your surgery you can start doing easy exercise. Such as leg lifts, shoulder rolls, any sitting exercises, and you can continue walking too. You can just increase the distance. Once you're about a month down the road from your surgery, you'll be able to crank it up a notch. Some exercises you should be able to do at this point are water aerobics and cycling. After a few more months you should be able to move onto strength training. This includes yoga, squats, and lunges. You can try going to the gym or do a workout from home. Start out with something easy and work your way up. If you choose to go to the gym you can start out with a smaller pair of weights and make a workout routine. If you choose to stay at home, it can be as simple as having a yoga mat and some resistance bands.

With any post-op care, whether it's eating or exercising, please take it slow! It may seem like things are progressing way too slowly, but your body needs this time to get used to doing things again after all it's been through.

Chapter 5: Life After Surgery

The first few weeks after surgery you'll probably be a little sore and be on an all liquid diet. You'll start walking around even if it's for 5 minutes at a time. You shouldn't try to do anything more physically demanding than that. Even a few months after surgery you'll still need to take it easy. You'll be eating more solid foods at this point and able to do more physically. At 6 months after surgery you'll have had a bit of weight loss. If you had gastric bypass surgery, then you will have lost 30%-40% of your excess weight. With gastric band surgery you lose about 1-2 pounds a week, so at this point would be anywhere from 25-50 pounds lost. One year after surgery you will have lost a significant amount of weight. The most dramatic changes happen within a year of your surgery. You are likely to your goal weight. With gastric banding you will have lost 100 pounds. If you haven't lost this amount it's important that you find the cause and make sure you are doing everything you can to contribute to your weight loss.

There are some changes you'll need to make with your personal life too after surgery if you wish to be successful with your weight loss journey. You'll need to tell your friends and family that it's very important for you to eat healthy from now on and stick to your smaller portions. It's much easier to stick to a healthy lifestyle when you have the support from everyone around you. But it can be that much harder if they don't. If your spouse, friends and family are still eating unhealthy and large portions then that can be really difficult to keep up with your healthy lifestyle. It's even possible that some people in your life might be jealous of you and might try to make you feel bad when you start to lose weight and they are still overweight. You should surround yourself with a group of people that support you and make it easier for you to live your new, healthy lifestyle. Losing weight can have a lot of impact on the relationships in your life. Hopefully for the better, but not always. How your relationship with your significant other if affected can depend a lot on how the relationship was before surgery. Did you have a good relationship? Was it not so good? If it was a bad relationship, they may have made you feel bad for being obese or maybe they liked your old weight and don't want you to change. If this is the case, they may become controlling and overly jealous when they see you losing weight. If you had a good relationship, then it should only strengthen your bond. If your S.O. decides to get healthier with you then that's great! If you have children then this choice will affect them too, but for the better! If you have a younger child, then you will help them develop healthy eating patterns and get used to eating healthy foods. If you have an older child, maybe even one that is overweight themselves, then you can help them make the changes earlier on in their life that you are now.

Chapter 6: How to Maintain Your Body and Stay in Shape

You'll have to learn how to take care of your new body. Not just right after surgery, but for the rest of your life. You'll have to be consistent in eating healthy and exercising if you want to stay in shape, you're going to have a whole lifestyle change! To stay consistent with working out, you should find a workout routine that works for you. Don't try to make yourself do something that you don't like to do. If you aren't a runner, try swimming. If you don't like lifting weights, try calisthenics. Find something that you can see yourself enjoying and progressing in. Plan your workout for the next few days in advance or every Sunday/Monday plan your workouts for the week ahead. You'll need to make a workout plan that you'll stick with. Set simple and easy to reach goals the first time around. Don't try to accomplish too much or you could hurt yourself or give up too early when you don't finish what you planned to. I know you're excited about losing weight and you want to get started, but you are more likely to lose less weight by planning to do more than you can actually accomplish. It's great to have big goals and you should always strive to progress and push past your limits to reach your new goal, but when you bite off more than you can chew you can't swallow! In other words, it's very easy to get discouraged in the beginning if you set impossible goals for yourself. It may take some time to see results in the beginning and that can be really hard to deal with. You're putting in so much work and you don't get to see any results yet. Believe me, if you push past this hump you WILL see results and by then you will have developed a habit eating healthy and working out. It will be so much easier to remain consistent once you do this. You've overcome the hardest obstacle, it is now a habit for you, and you've started to see results! Seeing the results that you've worked so hard for is the best motivation that you could receive.

Keeping a healthy diet is another goal you'll want to make sure you're reaching. Planning your meals ahead of time is a great way to avoid sneaking in snacks, overeating and binging an unhealthy meal. It takes the guesswork out of cooking and it'll probably save you from splurging at the grocery store. I would suggest planning your 3 big meals everyday and then also prepare for 2 healthy snacks a day. One in between breakfast and lunch, and one in between lunch and dinner. For your meals you should come up with an entrée, and for your sides and snacks you should make an approved healthy list to pick from. This list can of course grow if you find any snacks or sides you would like to try that are healthy. It's your choice if you wish to only prepare for the meal or if you would like to meal prep. Meal prepping is helpful because you don't have to put any thought into what you eat after it's prepped for the week because they are completely planned out, cooked, and ready for you to grab when it's time to eat. But if you like to cook or just don't want to cook all of your meals the next few days or week then you can stick to only planning what you're going to eat. You'll still have to make your food, but this is still helpful by taking the guesswork out of what you're going to eat. You shouldn't have any snacks after dinner because you are probably winding down for the day which means you aren't using as much energy from your body as you would in the middle of the day. Calories put into your body that aren't used will be stored and then turned into fat. Stick to liquids after dinner that way if you feel snacky you can drink some tea or water and you won't be putting very many, if any, calories in your body but your stomach will feel fuller.

Once you get started in your new lifestyle you will eventually need to progress past what you're doing now. Set new goals the same way you did your first ones. This time you are more acquainted with what you can accomplish which will allow you to set goals that will push you, but not set a goal that is unreachable. Although you should set goals that are realistically within your reach, you should never let anything get too easy and never let yourself get bored. That can go for more than just working out. You should try new things and create new challenges for yourself. Goals don't have to only be fitness related, they can be anything that helps to improve any part of your life. Your goals could include starting a new happy or progress in your job. There are so many things that we can do with life, you should never get bored! If you don't know what to do, that itself could be your goal. To go out and discover what you like. Maybe you have a creative side you never knew about. You could start writing, drawing, painting, or try out photography. Maybe you want to meet new people and make friends, or maybe you want to travel. There is so much out in the world to do that there should never be a reason to be bored. This is a great way to have a happy and healthy lifestyle before or after surgery. Staying busy and doing things that you love with people you care about can help depression, prevent overeating and unhealthy eating since you are staying busy, all of these things will help you overcome obesity.

Surgery or not, a big step in staying healthy and fit is consistency. It's going to be very hard for your body to lose weight if you aren't keeping up with your workouts and eating healthy. Pick a meal plan and a workout routine that fits your wants and needs and works with your schedule. Since your whole day is already planned it takes out any of the guesswork. You have a whole plan laid out you just have to go out and do it. Since you were productive, you'll feel happy and accomplished at the end of the day.

CONCLUSION

Good job for making it through to the end of the book. We hope it was informative and able to provide you with all of the tools you need to achieve your goals whatever they may be.

The next step is to put everything that you have learned in this book into practice. Learning more about your body and how it works is always a great place to start and in this book, we learned all about the acid-alkaline balance in our bodies, how the chemistry works, and what are the effects this balance or imbalance can have on our health.

We learned about some of the cutting edge science behind our understanding of pH levels in our body, and how we can fine tune them to the perfect level through our diet and other important practices. The human body is a very complicated and delicate machine, but the more we come to understand it, the better off we are and the more educated we can be in our choices regarding our health and wellbeing.

Given that your acid reflux is likely to exist on a ranging spectrum and will most definitely be different for every individual, this book provides methods of addressing your symptoms and ailments in a manner that is applicable and helpful for whichever stage of the reflux you are experiencing. What's more, the 30-day recovery plan is a great way to ensure that your symptoms are staved off for good once you can utilize medical intervention. If, for instance, you are prescribed drugs to mitigate your symptoms, be sure to use the methods outlined in this book in conjunction with the prescribed amount of medication that your doctor has instructed.

Where your health is concerned, being prepared and informed is critical to seeing that you successfully overcome the ailments that are affecting you.

That is precisely why this book is of value. After reading, you are now informed about the intricate aspects of acid reflux and should feel extremely prepared as you move forward in addressing these symptoms.

Now, it's up to you to take what you have learned in the preceding chapters and apply them into your life. Do you have what it takes to be in full control of your own health and get the very most out of your body? Will you settle for a body that works within tolerable levels, or do you want to maintain peak balance in your life and in your health? Then now is the time to apply all that you have learned and prove it for yourself!

Choose some of the recipes that appeal to you and start cooking! If you have completed your bariatric surgery, please be sure that you follow all post-operative instructions from your doctor or surgeon. If you have yet to complete your surgery, then take this time to try out a few of the recipes in this book and choose your favorites. You can go grocery shopping and be stocked up on all of the ingredients you will need after your surgery. You might even decide to cook ahead of time and make some freezer meals that will be easy to reheat after your surgery is complete. After your weight loss surgery, you will be making a complete lifestyle change. To that end, all of the recipes are suitable for meal prepping and can benefit you in packing breakfasts, lunches, and snacks that you can take along with you if you go to work or school.

So now you know all about Bariatric surgery. The different kinds of procedures and how they differ, how to prepare for it and what recovery will be like. If you are just starting out and trying to get information, I hope this helped you and once again congrats on taking the first step to a new and healthier life. If you are preparing for surgery, I hope this has helped you with your preparations and can make you feel more secure knowing what to expect on the day of your procedure. If you are currently in recovery, then this should have helped you with your diet and physical restrictions and what you are capable of doing right now. This book should also have given you an estimate of how much weight you can expect to lose from each type of procedure. Please keep in mind that any weight loss surgery can only help you to lose weight. You must be the one who wants to change and follow through with your plans. Surgery is not going to change your lifestyle, habits, addictions or any other cause of your obesity.

The next step is to put everything that you have learned in this book into practice. Learning more about your body and how it works is always a great place to start and in this book, we learned all about the acid-alkaline balance in our bodies, how the chemistry works, and what are the effects this balance or imbalance can have on our health.

We learned about some of the cutting edge science behind our understanding of pH levels in our body, and how we can fine tune them to the perfect level through our diet and other important practices. The human body is a very complicated and delicate machine, but the more we come to understand it, the better off we are and the more educated we can be in our choices regarding our health and wellbeing.

Now, it's up to you to take what you have learned in the preceding chapters and apply them into your life. Do you have what it takes to be in full control of your own health and get the very most out of your body? Will you settle for a body that works within tolerable levels, or do you want to maintain peak balance in your life and in your health? Then now is the time to apply all that you have learned and prove it for yourself!